YOGA

— FOR —

COMMON AILMENTS

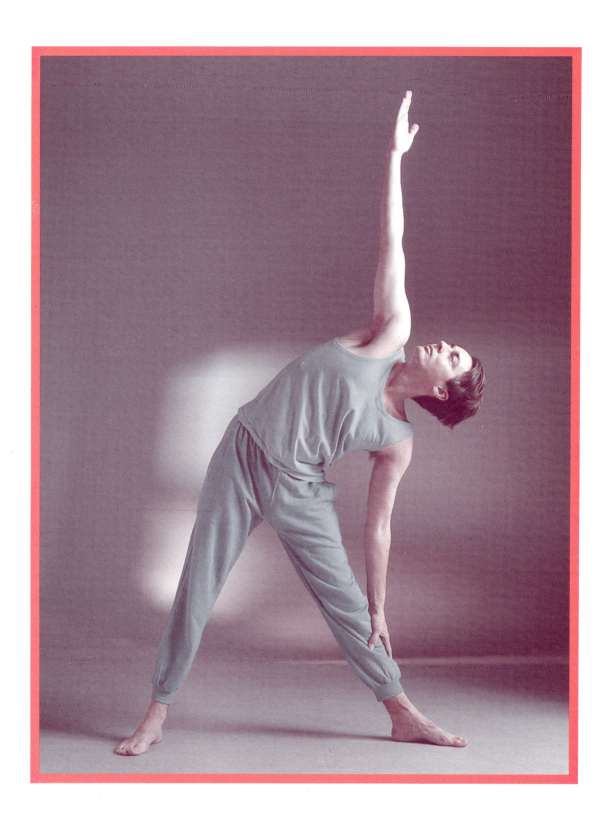

YOGA

—— FOR ——

COMMON AILMENTS

Dr R Nagarathna · Dr H R Nagendra · Dr Robin Monro

Based on the system developed by the
Vivekananda Kendra Yoga Research Foundation
(Bangalore, H Q Kanyakumari, India)

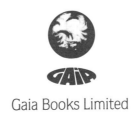

Gaia Books Limited

A GAIA ORIGINAL

Based on an idea by Lucy Lidell

Based on the system developed by the
Vivekananda Kendra Yoga Research Foundation
(Bangalore, H Q Kanyakumari, India)

Written by	Dr R Nagarathna Dr H R Nagendra Dr Robin Monro
Editorial	Eve Webster
Design	Helen Spencer
Illustrations	Sheilagh Noble
Photography	Fausto Dorelli
Production	Susan Walby
Direction	Jonathan Hilton Joss Pearson

® This is a Registered Trade Mark
of Gaia Books Limited

First published in the United Kingdom by
Gaia Books Limited
66 Charlotte Street
London W1P 1LR

British Library Cataloguing in Publication Data
Nagarathna, R
    Yoga for common ailments.
    1. Man. Therapy. Use of yoga
    I. Title II. Nagendra, H.R. III. Monro, Robin
    615.89

ISBN 1-85675-010-8

Publisher's Acknowledgements
Gaia would like to extend special thanks
to the following: Dr David Clark, Nancy
Ford-Kohne, Lesley Gilbert, Michele Staple,
Libby Hoseason, Lynette Beckford, Sara
Mathews, Louise Grime, Dominique Radclyffe,
Simon de Wrangel, Penelope Barton, Subhadra
Devi, Tewani Mohan, On Yer Bike, and
Federal Express.

The techniques, ideas, and suggestions in this
book are not intended as a substitute for proper
medical advice. Consult your physician or health
care professional before beginning this or any
new exercise program, particularly if you are
pregnant or nursing, or if you are elderly or
if you have any chronic or recurring physical
conditions. Any application of the techniques,
ideas, and suggestions in this book is at the
reader's sole discretion and risk.

Typeset by Tradespools Limited, Somerset, UK.
Reproduction by Fotographics, London, UK.
Printed and bound by Mateu Cromo, Madrid, Spain.

Information on the Centres

In 1975 Dr H R Nagendra gave up a prestigious and successful career in engineering in order to work for the Vivekananda Yoga Centre. Shortly afterward he established the Vivekananda Kendra Yoga Research Foundation (VYF) in Bangalore, South India, of which he became full-time director. The aim of VYF was to bring the benefits of yoga into daily life and to carry out critical research into the effectiveness of yoga therapy. Dr Nagendra was helped in this task by Dr R Nagarathna, who qualified in internal medicine and is a member of the Royal College of Physicians in Edinburgh. She provided the medical know-how needed to develop the Vivekananda system of yoga therapy, which is also used in this book. She now works at the centre as a consulting yoga therapist.

VYF has trained hundreds of yoga therapists, helped thousands of people with chronic disorders, and has carried out critical research into the effectiveness of yoga therapy for bronchial asthma, diabetes mellitus, and several other ailments. It has published the results in the *British Medical Journal* and other medical journals. At its base near Bangalore, it has a hospital, and a research centre, and runs training courses for yoga therapists and for school teachers. It also carries out training and research programmes in the USA, the UK, and Japan.

Robin Monro is a board member of the World Federation of Societies of Holistic Medicine, a board member of Unity in Yoga, and a board member of the International Association of Yoga Therapists, as well as being the full-time director of the Yoga Biomedical Trust. Originally, he studied biochemistry at Cambridge University and then spent 12 years on basic research into protein biosynthesis. He became concerned, however, over the broader cultural issues raised by developments in the biosciences. This led him to focus on holistic medicine as a field in which philosophical, ethical, and scientific issues intersect.

He established the Yoga Biomedical Trust (YBT) in Cambridge, UK, in 1983. The aim of the Trust is to promote research into, and the practice of, yoga therapy. With its Advisory Council of eminent doctors and scientists, and in collaboration with several different yoga organizations, YBT seeks to explore, freely and critically, the therapeutic potentials of yoga. So far, the surveys it has carried out suggest that people who take up yoga are helped with a wide variety of ailments, visit the doctor less often, and take less sick leave. It is also carrying out clinical trials of yoga for premenstrual syndrome, headaches, and fibromyalgia, and collaborating with the Vivekananda Kendra Yoga Research Foundation to do trials on diabetes mellitus and rheumatoid arthritis. The Trust also maintains an information service on yoga therapy, and runs a training course for yoga therapists in conjunction with the Vivekananda Kendra Yoga Research Foundation.

CONTENTS

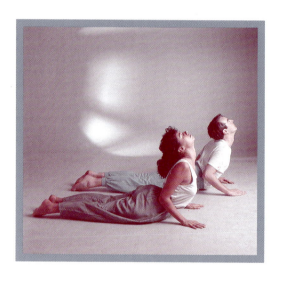

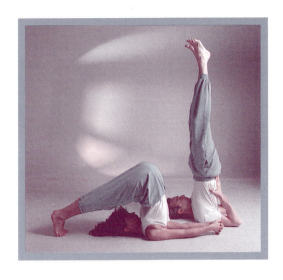

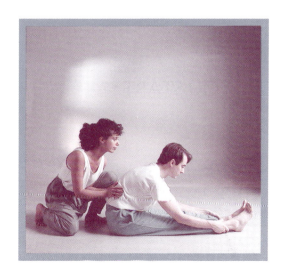

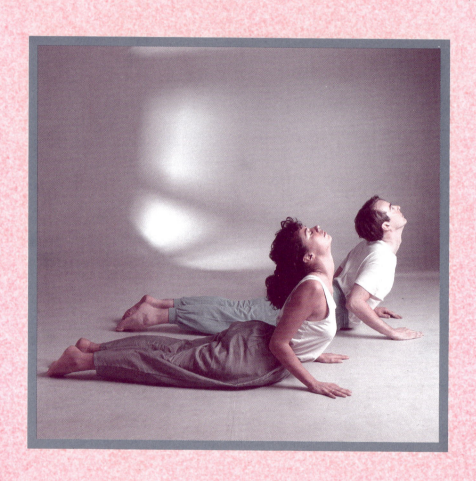

INTRODUCTION

"Yoga is skill in action" states the *Bhagavad Gita*, the best known of all the Indian philosophical epics. But this is not intended to mean action in just the narrow sense of physical movement. For as well as exercises for improving the "skill" of your body, yoga also comprises techniques that act on your mind and emotions, and provides a complete philosophy for living.

In order to achieve this aim you must develop "skill" in all aspects of your life. A great Indian teacher of this century, Sri Aurobindo, regarded yoga as a methodical effort toward self-perfection through developing your latent potential on the physical, vital, mental, intellectual, and spiritual levels. And the most fundamental step you can take toward expanding the limits of your consciousness is to gain mastery over your mind.

This is also the key to good health and happiness in today's world. Great advances in medical science over the past century have reduced the incidence of most of the physical diseases that have plagued humanity for centuries. Ever-better drugs and surgical techniques have led to the eradication of most infectious diseases and the control of many metabolic disorders. Soon even routine genetic interventions may be possible. But these techniques are less than effective against the new and ever-more-common causes of ill health – chronic stress and psychosomatic ailments.

Conventional medicine, by concentrating on a physical and mechanistic approach to healing, can do little to relieve conditions such as these, since they are caused more by lifestyle and attitudes than by physiological anomalies. The frenetic pace of modern life exposes many people to continuous, unrelieved stress. And if you are largely sedentary in your habits and overindulge in health-damaging substances and foods, your wellbeing and fitness will be further compromised. Eventually stress may manifest itself in the form of physical disease or mental breakdown. Modern medicine has countered with symptom-suppressing treatments, which do little to tackle the root cause of the problem. As a result, health has come to be regarded as a static state in which disease is absent, rather than as a dynamic growth process in which you feel truly *well* on both the physical and mental levels. But there is no reason to settle for anything less than a positive sense of wellbeing.

Yoga has a lot to offer as we approach the 21st century. It gives us the means to complement medical technology with a holistic system of healthcare that addresses the problems of the mind and spirit, as well as those of the body. Patanjali, who wrote the classic text on yoga more than 2000 years ago, described it as "a science of the mind". And it is through teaching you to control your mind, your desires, and your reactions to stress that yoga can fundamentally help you.

Mastery of the mind involves two aspects: the ability to concentrate your attention on any given subject or object; and the capacity to quieten your mind at will. Though most people have developed the first aspect to some degree, extremely few of us can lapse into inner peace even accidentally, let alone at will. Yoga is an intelligent, skilful means for making the mind quiet, rather than a brutal, mechanical technique for stopping it.

All aspects of yoga work toward this in some way, thus bringing you closer to your goal. Yoga develops your ability to maintain inner peace at all times, in all your actions, and thereby achieve physical and mental health. This calmness in action is the secret to attaining the "skill" referred to in the *Bhagavad Gita*.

YOGA AND HEALTH

The approach of yoga therapy is based on ancient Indian traditional beliefs about human existence. In this philosophy there are five "sheaths" to existence, as shown in the illustration on page 12, of which the physical frame is only the first. The second is the vital body that is made up of *prana*, the life energy that flows through you in invisible channels known as *nadis*. The third is the mind (your emotions and thoughts), the fourth is the higher intellect (perfect thought and knowledge), and the final sheath is the "abode of bliss". The bliss sheath is thought to consist of the positive energy that is associated with the divine. It is from this sheath that the inner peace essential to true happiness emanates.

Disease is seen to arise through imbalance in any of the three lower sheaths of existence. In the physical, *pranic*, and mind sheaths, ego consciousness, which is centred around the self, predominates and therefore harmony in these sheaths can be easily disturbed. The fourth and fifth sheaths are permeated by a wider, universal consciousness and cannot be perturbed. When you are truly healthy, the positive energy in the highest sheath percolates freely through the lower ones and brings total harmony and balance to all your faculties. But though the harmony of the higher sheaths is constant, the free movement of bliss can be blocked by imbalances in the lower sheaths.

The concept of the five sheaths is not entirely accepted by Western science but it is relevant from an experiential viewpoint. In time, it is possible to "feel" both *prana* and bliss without knowing whether they are independent energies or simply the expression of complex physiological phenomena. And by "feeling" and manipulating *prana*, yogis achieve a remarkable control over their bodies that can readily be confirmed by scientific tests. Accordingly, in this book such concepts are referred to as if they exist even though objective proof is lacking

In Indian philosophy there are two types of physical illness, and each requires a different approach. The first are the illnesses with a strong physical element, such as contagious diseases and accidental injuries. These are most effectively dealt with by conventional medicine, though yoga can play a substantial supporting role. Yoga also helps prevent the occurrence of such ailments by improving your general health and making you less accident-prone.

The other type of illness arises through disturbances in the mind sheath and includes all the psychosomatic and degenerative ailments. In these disorders, psychological factors play a much greater role, and conventional treatment alone is not usually an effective cure. According to Indian beliefs, such ailments are thought to be caused by mental diseases called *adhis*. These arise when excessively strong feelings of like or dislike become amplified and established, acting to distort personality and to obstruct the flow of positive energy to the lower sheaths. This causes imbalances that result in physical ailments and also makes you feel restless and discontent.

The inner peace that is your natural state is generated by the positive energy from the "bliss" sheath. When the flow of this energy is interrupted by *adhis*, your sense of wellbeing is diminished and, in your attempt to regain it, you may be further aggravating the problem by behaving inappropriately. You may, for example, find yourself eating the wrong foods, living in unhealthy surroundings, lapsing into negative states of mind, or driving yourself too hard. But these methods give only temporary relief and may, in fact, be damaging your health.

With psychosomatic ailments, yoga provides the vital element that modern therapies lack and acts directly on the mental imbalances that underlie them. While *Emotion Culturing* and *Meditation* make you aware of

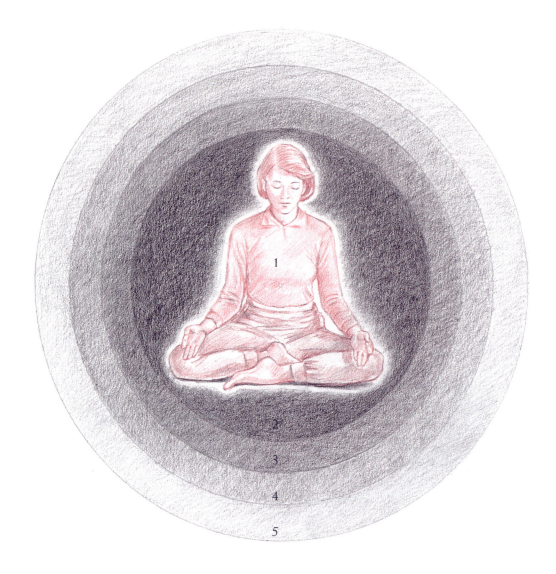

THE FIVE SHEATHS OF EXISTENCE

Each successive sheath includes
and transcends those inside it.
The outermost is beyond time and space.

1 Physical body
2 Vital body (*prana*)
3 Mind (lower mental)
4 Intellect (higher mental)
5 Bliss (universal consciousness)

the tyranny of thoughts and emotions, *Happiness Analysis* teaches you how to look within yourself to find peace and satisfaction. At the same time, other yoga practices facilitate the restoration of health at other levels as well. This effectively complements medical techniques, which improve the situation physically but are unable to eradicate the primary cause of the problem.

HAPPINESS ANALYSIS

This involves trying to understand the nature of bliss, the inner peace that characterizes the fifth level of being. It basically embodies the realization that happiness comes from within and is not dependent on material possessions or physical enjoyment.

Happiness is often associated with jubilance and excitement, or the satisfaction of achieving desires. But these sources of pleasure are temporary, and in receding they are often followed by negative feelings, such as tiredness or disillusionment. Real, sustainable inner peace involves no effort and engenders no fatigue. The texts of yoga describe complete happiness as a state of silence, where you are no longer troubled by unnecessary thoughts and fears, a state of perfect poise and freedom of choice.

Yogic practices lay the foundation needed for you to achieve this, but you must also try to identify consciously what perfect happiness is and attempt to cultivate and maintain such a state for as long as you can. Start by analysing what the feeling of pleasure comprises as you do something you enjoy. Yogis claim that actions bring pleasure when they briefly evoke the inner silence that defines true happiness. At the moment when you obtain something you desire or attain a hard-won goal – at the very instance of success – your thoughts vanish and your mind dips momentarily into the sheath of "bliss". This is the source of pleasure and all likes and dislikes – certain actions, or experiences, tend to open up temporary channels to the higher sheath, hence evoking positive sensations. But this feeling is temporary, and can tempt us to overindulge in the activity or substance that generated it.

If you can isolate and remember that brief moment of satisfaction, however, you can learn to generate it from within and free yourself from dependency on external aids. At first you may not be able to maintain inner peace for long, but gradually you will become less vulnerable to negative influences. The likes and dislikes that can lead to *adhis* (p. 11) will become less important and your growing awareness of universal consciousness will give meaning and coherence to every aspect of your life.

THE BASIS OF YOGA THERAPY

Yoga is fundamentally different from conventional medical practice in its approach to healthcare. Instead of trying to reduce the cause of disease to a single factor and to correct it using a specific cure, yoga aims to treat illness by improving health on all levels simultaneously and by restoring inner harmony.

Ill health occurs when the total balance of perfect health is disturbed (pp. 10-11). And although the original disrupting influence may only affect one level at first, the disturbance soon spreads. All the five sheaths of existence interact, thus something that primarily affects the mind, say, can soon spread to the body and *pranic* sheaths. A bad day at work may make you irritable, for example, but it also increases stress reactions, it may make you tense your muscles, and often depletes your energy level, leading to chronic fatigue.

For this reason, yoga contains elements that address problems at every level – *asanas* that relax and tone your muscles and massage your internal organs, *pranayama* that slows breathing and regulates the flow of *prana*, relaxation and meditation that act to calm your mind, and emotion culturing to heal your spirit. For just as negative influences spread disruption, positive action has repercussions as well. The different types of yoga practice augment each other and are more effective when done together. When you do the *asanas* and stretch your muscles, muscular tension is released and you are more able to relax. Likewise, when you relax the mind and release suppressed emotions you tend to become less tense on a physical level. Every element of yoga brings benefits throughout, and also acts to amplify the effect of the other types of practices.

This is the essence of yoga therapy – both as a preventive and as a curative. Daily practice of a complete yoga session can restore your natural balance and harmony, bringing positive good health to all parts of your life – physical, mental, and spiritual.

HOW TO USE THIS BOOK

Yoga for Common Ailments shows you how to design and practise a daily yoga session, both to preserve your health and to aid recovery from specific ailments. Part 1, on pages 16-43, outlines the *Basic Session*, a general programme to improve health and fitness. Unless you have a specific ailment, you need only look at Part 1.

If you plan to use yoga as part of a therapy programme for a particular condition, you may need to modify the *Basic Session*. With chronic or severe ailments, some yoga practices can be dangerous and should be avoided. In others, recovery may be hastened by changing the emphasis and contents of your daily session. Hence, *The Ailments* section, on pages 44-91, shows you how to design an ailment-specific session for many common conditions. It explains the cause of the ailment and how yoga can help, and also gives general advice and cautions. At the end of each ailment there is an "advice box" (where applicable) that shows you how to modify the *Basic Session*. This lists the exercises that you should give more time to, or "emphasize", the ones that you should avoid, and also suggests additional practices that will be beneficial to you but are not included in the *Basic Session* as part of the general purpose yoga programme.

First read page 45, which gives detailed instructions on how to design an individual programme. Then read the advice given for your ailment. For easy reference the ailments are separated into sections, each dealing with a major body system (see Contents). In some cases, however, where the yoga session for a number of ailments is similar, two or more ailments may be dealt with under one major heading. Therefore, if you cannot find the disorder you wish to treat, try looking for it in the index (pp. 92-4).

Having done this go back and read pages 16-19 for advice on how to plan and time your yoga session and pages 20-43 for instructions on how to do the exercises. Even though you may have to modify the *Basic Session* in order to tailor it to your ailment, never lose sight of the holistic approach that defines yoga therapy (p. 14). You will obtain no benefit by practising only the exercises that have been recommended for your ailment and omitting all the rest. Retain as much of the programme as you can, only omitting those parts that you are specifically warned against.

Finally, always bear in mind that although yoga and the special programmes in this book can bring you great benefits, they are not designed as a substitute for conventional medical care. Always consult your doctor in addition to using yogic therapies and never use this book for self-diagnosis. Yoga cannot totally replace modern therapies and in many cases surgery or drugs may be necessary to avoid serious ill health. Rather, modern medicine and ancient yogic therapies should be used in conjunction with one another. In this way, yoga can maximize the effectiveness of modern treatments and alleviate their more serious side-effects. It may, for example, allow you to reduce your dosage of drugs, if this is agreed to by a health care professional. Best of all, yoga gives you the means to promote your health and wellbeing actively – long before you need to go to the doctor.

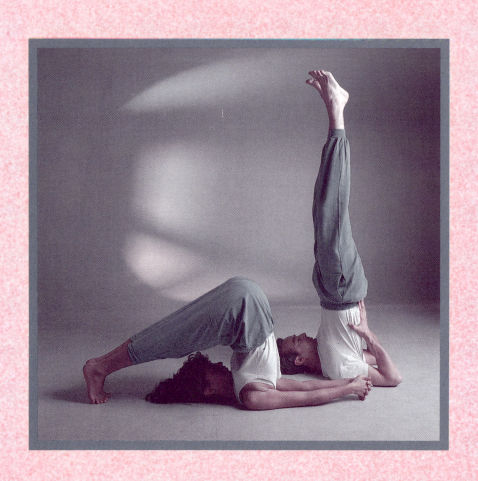

THE BASIC SESSION

Yoga is a way of living – a means of achieving health in body, mind, and spirit. For it to be effective, however, you must make it a part of your life and practise daily. The *Basic Session*, on pages 18–43, provides a framework on which to base your daily yoga session.

The *Basic Session* exercises are laid out in the order that you should do them. The preliminary exercises in *Before You Start* prepare you for the *asanas* and also act to calm you. The four cycles of *asanas* that follow are ordered in "counterposes" so that each group counterbalances the one before. This is followed by *Relaxation* then by breathing practices in *Pranayama* and the session ends with *Meditation*. *Emotion Culturing* and *Diet and Lifestyle* explain how to introduce the health-sustaining yogic way in your everyday dealings.

Pages 18–19 show you how to rotate certain practices in order to construct a realistic general session. Advice on how to make an ailment-specific session is given in *The Ailments* (pp. 44–91). Go to a qualified yoga teacher to learn yoga if you can, especially if you are using this book to aid treatment. And consult a doctor or yoga specialist if you have an ailment not mentioned in this book.

Find a quiet place for your yoga session, either out of doors or in a tidy, well-ventilated room. Wear loose, comfortable clothing and place a mat or blanket on the floor to make yourself more comfortable. Avoid bright lights, and distractions or interruptions.

GENERAL CAUTIONS

While the practices in this book are gentle and safe, it is not possible to cover all eventualities. Always consult your doctor or a yoga specialist if you feel uncertain about a particular technique. Use extreme caution if you have a serious health problem or have had any kind of surgery. If you are pregnant, avoid all exercises in *Before You Start* (pp. 20–5), all forward bending, *Rapid Abdominal Breathing* (p. 39), *Abdominal Lock* (p. 74), *Abdominal Pumping* (p. 76), *Forced Alternate-nostril Breathing* (p. 70), and *Prone Asanas* (pp. 29–30). Spend more time on *DRT* (p. 37), *Pranayama* (pp. 38–9), and *Meditation* (p. 40). After the twelfth week of pregnancy avoid all *Asanas* (pp. 26–35). A simplified session with modified *asanas*, designed by a yoga specialist, can be useful.

HOW TO PLAN YOUR DAILY SESSION

The effectiveness of yoga depends on frequent, regular practice, even if only for a short period each day. To achieve this, you need an efficient session that covers your needs, and you will have to make a realistic assessment of your abilities and the time you can spare. To design an ailment-specific yoga session, first read page 45 and the section on the ailment you suffer from. When you have done this, or if you only need a general programme to promote and preserve your health, you can then work out when, what, and how long you need to practise every day.

Establish a regular time for your session, either before breakfast or before your evening meal. If this is not possible, wait at least an hour after a snack and three and a half hours after a main meal before starting. Choose either the long (one-hour) or short (half-hour) version of the *Basic Session* (see chart). In both cases, some exercises will have to be rotated over two-day intervals, as shown by the symbols on the chart. If time is extremely short, you need only practise the *Sun Salute*.

Ailment-specific sessions may last longer than an hour because they often contain additional and "emphasize" exercises. To make them shorter, rotate the rest of the practices over several days. In this case bear in mind that each session should contain a bend in every direction and that if you twist or stretch in one way you should also do the same in the opposite direction. This is the principle of "counterposes".

Practise what suits you and your needs. Everyone's capacities differ, so you should not ignore your own preferences. But neither should you ignore the cautions given in the *Ailments* section, unless you first seek professional advice. In general, start with the practices that you find easy, and gradually incorporate the more difficult ones. The chart gives some guidelines that will help you decide what to try first and, as you improve, you can add more. But do not try to progress too quickly; it is far better to learn slowly and well.

USING THE CHART

The exercises are listed in the order that you should do them. Some of these may be marked with an asterisk (*), in which case you should avoid them until you are confident that you have mastered the easier practices. The second column contains symbols showing you which exercises to rotate on alternate days. Exercises marked with ■ should all be done on one day, and exercises marked with □ on the following day. When an exercise has both symbols you should do it every day. The third column gives the times for the long daily session and the fourth column for the shorter version. The last column gives *maximum* times that you can aim toward when you are asked to "emphasize" exercises; but do not strain to achieve these from the start.

	Exercises	Rotating Exercises 1	Rotating Exercises 2	Time (minutes) Full session	Short session	Emphasize
BREATHE AND STRETCH	**BEFORE YOU START**					
	Arm-stretch Breathing	□	■	1	½	2
	Hand-stretch Breathing	□	■	2	—	2
	Tree Breathing	□	■	1	—	1½
	Cat Stretch	□	■	1	½	2
	Rabbit Breathing	□	■	½	—	½
	Single-leg Raising	□	■	2	1½	2
LOOSENING UP AND SUN SALUTE	Jogging	□	■	2	1	2
	Forward-backward Bending	□	■	½	½	½
	Sideways Bending	□	■	½	—	½
	Twisting	□	■	½	½	½
	Embryo	□	■	1	—	1
	Sun Salute*	□	■ ○	3½	1½	10
	Instant Relaxation Technique	□	■	2	2	2
STANDING	**ASANAS**					
	Lateral Arc	□		4	4	4
	Hands-to-feet Pose	□		3	3	3
	Backward Bend	□		2	2	2
	Triangle*	□		½	—	½
PRONE	Cobra		■	2	1	4
	Locust		■	2	1	4
	Bow*		■	1	½	3
	Crocodile		■	1	½	3
SUPINE	Half Shoulderstand or		■	2	2	5
	Shoulderstand*		■	2	2	5
	Plough*		■	1	—	3
	Bridge		■	1	—	3
	Fish*		■	1	1	3
SITTING	Kneeling Pose	□		1	½	2
	Moon	□		2	—	3
	Camel*	□		2	—	3
	Spinal Twist		■	3	—	4
	Forward Stretch		■	2	1	4
	Supine Kneebend*		■	1	—	4
RELAX-ATION	**RELAXATION**					
	Quick Relaxation Technique (QRT) or	□	■	5	5	10
	Deep Relaxation Technique (DRT)	□	■	10	5	20
PRANAYAMA AND MEDITATION	**PRANAYAMA & MEDITATION**					
	Sectional Breathing	□	■	4	1	5
	Rapid Abdominal Breathing*	□	■	4	2	10
	Alternate-nostril Breathing*	□	■	4	2	10
	Folded-tongue Breathing*		■	1		2
	Sounds Breathing	□		2	—	3
	Meditation		■	5	5	15

□ = Rotating exercises Day 1   ○ = Can omit from general session
■ = Rotating exercises Day 2   * = Difficult exercises

BEFORE YOU START

BREATHE AND STRETCH
The gentle exercises on this page cultivate the mental state you need to practise yoga. Close your eyes as you do them and be aware of your inner sensations. Always breathe out for longer than you breathe in, synchronizing your breathing and movement. Note how you become calmer as your breathing slows.
CAUTION ○ Avoid:
Cat Stretch for *epilepsy*
Rabbit Breathing for *epilepsy*

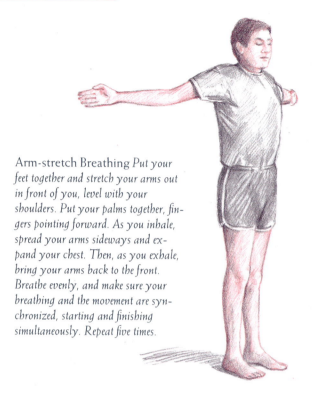

Arm-stretch Breathing *Put your feet together and stretch your arms out in front of you, level with your shoulders. Put your palms together, fingers pointing forward. As you inhale, spread your arms sideways and expand your chest. Then, as you exhale, bring your arms back to the front. Breathe evenly, and make sure your breathing and the movement are synchronized, starting and finishing simultaneously. Repeat five times.*

Hand-stretch Breathing *Stand upright and place your hands on your chest, with your fingers interlinked and palms facing inward. As you inhale, stretch out your arms horizontally to the position shown and reverse your hands so that the palms face outward. Bring them back to your chest as you exhale. Repeat three times. Then, do the same again, but now raise your arms to 45°, rather than extending them horizontally. Repeat again, raising your arms to the vertical, above your head.*

Tree Breathing *Stand upright, arms down and fingers interlocked, with your palms facing down. As you inhale, rise up on your toes, and at the same time bring your hands up to your chest, and on up, raising your arms above your head as in the final part of Hand-stretch Breathing. Feel the stretch from your ankles to your fingers as you reach upward. Then, as you exhale, lower your arms and go down on your heels again. Repeat five times.*

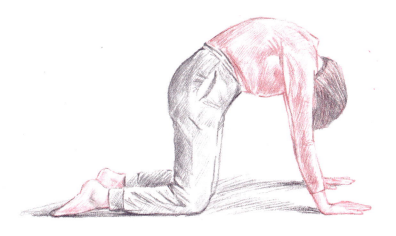

Cat Stretch *Crouch down on your hands and knees, with your arms and thighs vertical, like pillars. As you exhale, slowly lower your head and arch your back up, so that it is convex. Then, as you inhale, bend your head up and bring your spine down so that it is concave. Feel the stretch along your spine, neck, and shoulders. Repeat several times, breathing slowly, and accentuate the upward and downward stretches of the spine as much as possible – don't just move your head.*

Rabbit Breathing *Kneel down on the ground and sit back on your heels. Then, bend forward from the waist and rest your elbows and palms on the ground beside your knees. Your hands should be facing forward, and your head held up. Open your mouth, stick out your tongue, and pant quickly like a rabbit. Use only the upper part of the chest and continue for 20 breaths. Then close your mouth and sit up.*

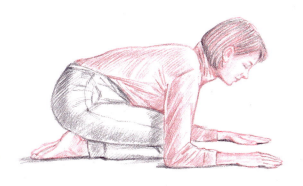

Single-leg Raising *Lie down, with your arms by your sides. As you inhale, slowly raise your right leg up, without bending your knee, as far as you can without feeling pain in your hamstrings. Then, exhale as you lower it. Keep your lower back close to the floor. Do five leg-raises for each leg. If this begins to be easy, also do* Double-leg Raising *(p. 58) after you finish, but note any cautions.*

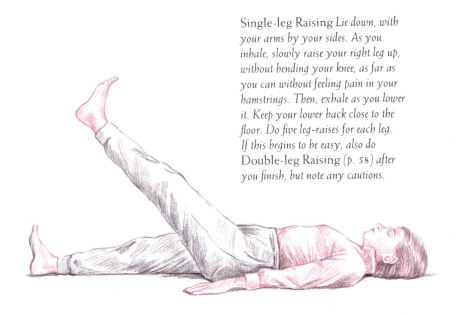

LOOSENING UP
These dynamic exercises prepare you for the *asanas*.
CAUTION ○ Avoid:
Loosening Up for hypertension, venous blood clots, heart disease, first month of yoga near menopause.
Jogging for varicose veins, back pain, haemorrhoids, hernia, disc problems.
Forward-backward Bending for low back pain, hernia, disc problems, glaucoma, pressure in head and neck.
Sideways Bending for low back pain, hernia, disc problems.
Twisting for hernia, disc problems.

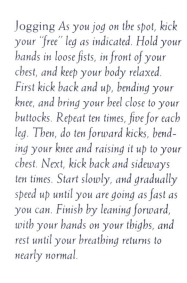

Jogging *As you jog on the spot, kick your "free" leg as indicated. Hold your hands in loose fists, in front of your chest, and keep your body relaxed. First kick back and up, bending your knee, and bring your heel close to your buttocks. Repeat ten times, five for each leg. Then, do ten forward kicks, bending your knee and raising it up to your chest. Next, kick back and sideways ten times. Start slowly, and gradually speed up until you are going as fast as you can. Finish by leaning forward, with your hands on your thighs, and rest until your breathing returns to nearly normal.*

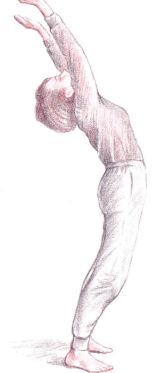

Forward-backward Bending
Inhaling, stretch your arms upward and backward and bend your spine back. Exhaling, come back up and then bend forward as far as you can. Repeat this forward/backward motion, inhaling as you go back and exhaling as you come forward. Gradually increase the speed and bring a swinging movement to the body and arms. Avoid excessive speed or jerking.

Sideways Bending *Stand with your feet wide apart. As you inhale, raise your right arm to your shoulder, parallel to the ground. Exhaling, bend to the left, sliding your left arm along your left thigh toward your heel; turn your head back and look along the line of your right arm, keeping your chin in and your body in one plane. Come up as you inhale. Then do the same on the right. Repeat ten times, five for each side. Start slowly, then gradually increase the speed after a few days.*

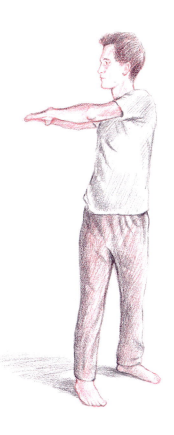

Twisting *Stand with your feet 60cm (24in) apart, and your arms spread out horizontally. As you exhale, twist to the right and extend your right arm back, bending your left arm at the elbow and looking behind you. Keep your body straight. Inhaling, turn to the front, and now twist to the left. Repeat many times, gradually increasing the speed and breathing rate. Take care not to jerk or strain.*

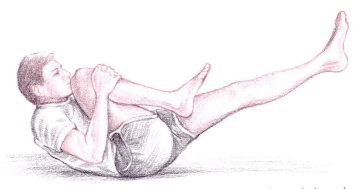

Embryo *Lie with your heels together, arms stretched out behind you. Bend your knees as you raise your legs, and inhale slowly. Then, as you exhale, tuck your knees in to your chest, holding them with interlocked fingers, and bring your chin up to your knees. Next, extend your left leg at 45° and rotate it in the air, five times clockwise and five times counterclockwise, breathing normally. Repeat, with your right. Finally, bring both legs to your chest and rock back and forth a few times.*

Instant Relaxation Technique (IRT) *Lie as shown and then, inhale and tighten your toes, feet, and calves, pull your kneecaps back, and clench your thighs and buttocks. Exhale, pulling in your abdomen, clenching your fists, and tightening the muscles in your arms. Inhale, expand your chest, and tighten your shoulders, neck, and facial muscles. Go on tightening your body for about three seconds, then release as you exhale, and spread your legs and arms. Let your body relax. Do not alter the order given above, and allow a few seconds for each muscle group.*

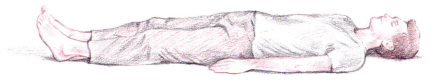

23

SUN SALUTE

In India this practice is traditionally performed at sunrise and sunset, facing the rising or setting sun. If this is not feasible, imagine a sunrise over a beautiful scene, bathing you in sunlight.

You can practise the *Sun Salute* on its own when you cannot do a long session. Do the rounds in pairs, one for each leg, and practise IRT (p. 23) at the end.

CAUTION ○ Avoid:
Sun Salute for hypertension, hernia, low back pain, venous blood clots.

11 *Exhaling, bring your left foot up beside your right. Then straighten both legs and reach down with your upper body. Inhaling, stand erect. Now you can either stop or repeat the cycle. Start each successive round with alternate legs.*

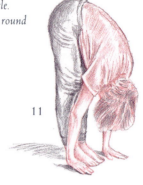

11

10

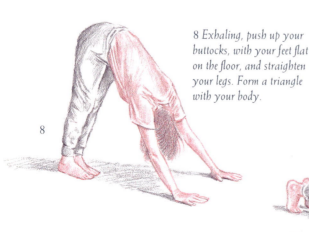

9

9 & 10 *Inhaling, bend your knees, resting your buttocks on your heels, forehead on the floor. Exhale, then inhaling, bring your right knee up between your hands.*

8 *Exhaling, push up your buttocks, with your feet flat on the floor, and straighten your legs. Form a triangle with your body.*

8

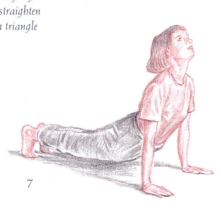

7 *Without inhaling, come forward, taking your weight on your hands, and rest your knees, chest, and forehead on the floor. But keep your abdomen off the ground. Then, inhaling, push up with your arms and stretch back your head to make your spine concave.*

7

24

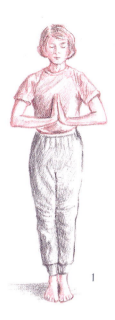

1 & 2 *Stand erect, with your feet together. Place your palms against each other, and hold them up to your chest, fingers pointing upward. Chant "OM HRAM" and then, as you inhale, raise your hands up above your head and bend back. Your palms should be facing up and your head should be reaching back.*

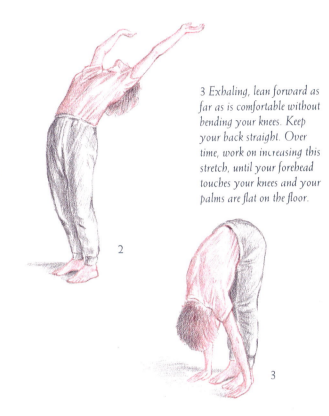

3 *Exhaling, lean forward as far as is comfortable without bending your knees. Keep your back straight. Over time, work on increasing this stretch, until your forehead touches your knees and your palms are flat on the floor.*

4 *As you inhale, bend your knees and put your palms flat on the ground beside your feet. Then, take your right leg back as far as you can, knee just resting on the floor. Look up, and push your hips forward.*

5 & 6 *Bring your left leg back, next to your right and exhale completely. Inhale as you go back, and rest your buttocks on your heels and your forehead on the floor. Then exhale.*

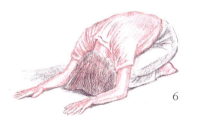

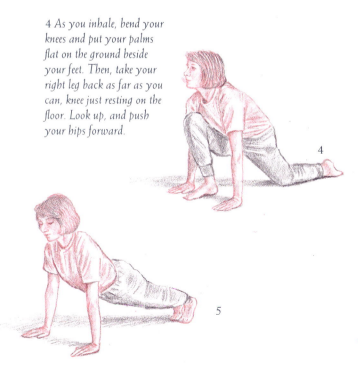

25

ASANAS

The yoga postures, or *asanas*, work at a much deeper level than the preceding exercises. They release your muscles and joints, and holding the postures tones your muscles, massages your internal organs, and promotes better breathing and circulation. On a more subtle level, the *asanas* also release the flow of energy within you, and relaxing your muscles acts to calm and still your mind.

As you do the *asanas*, be aware of the sensations in your body. Feel the stretches, the changes in pressure, and how your breathing slows down. Let yourself relax further into the *asanas* as you exhale, and hold the position you reach as you inhale. When you have mastered this, holding the postures will seem to need almost no effort. But until you reach this level of awareness, be extremely careful and make sure you do not hurt yourself. Try to minimize effort from the start, and if you are sensitive to your body you will soon learn the correct postures as you do them. Above all, do not strain in order to achieve the final position. Just find your natural limit for that stretch, where you feel comfortable, and slowly try to increase it from there.

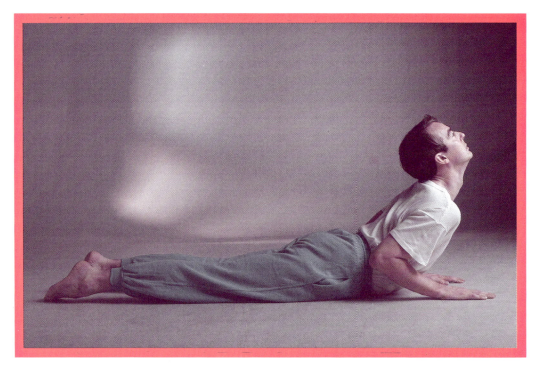

THE COBRA

STANDING ASANAS

This cycle of dynamic, standing positions strengthens your muscles, improves your balance, and gives your body a stretch in every direction. This prepares you for the *Prone, Supine,* and *Sitting Asanas* that follow.

CAUTION ○ Avoid:
Standing Asanas for *blood clots*
Hands-to-feet Pose for *hypertension, glaucoma, pressure in head and neck.*

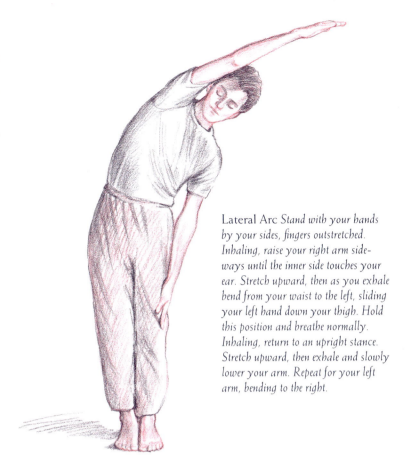

Lateral Arc *Stand with your hands by your sides, fingers outstretched. Inhaling, raise your right arm sideways until the inner side touches your ear. Stretch upward, then as you exhale bend from your waist to the left, sliding your left hand down your thigh. Hold this position and breathe normally. Inhaling, return to an upright stance. Stretch upward, then exhale and slowly lower your arm. Repeat for your left arm, bending to the right.*

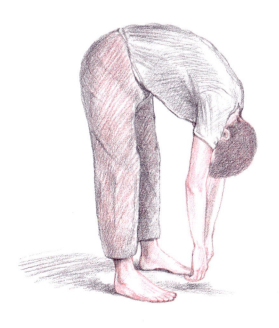

Hands-to-feet Pose *From standing, inhale and lift your arms sideways, until they are over your head. Stretch up from the base of your spine. Exhale and bend forward until your upper body is horizontal; also reach upward, keeping your back concave and bending at the hips. Inhale, then, exhaling, bend down. Let your back curve but still bend mostly from the hips. Go down as low as you can without straining or bending your legs, and hold this position. Then, inhaling, raise your upper body to the horizontal position. Exhale. Inhaling, raise yourself upright and exhale as you lower your arms.*

27

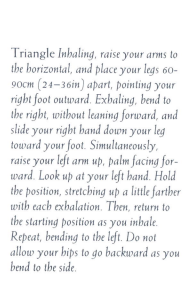

Backward Bend *From standing, slide your hands up to your waist, resting them on your hips with your fingers pointing forward. As you inhale, slowly bend backward from the middle of your body, stretching your head and neck back as well. If you have neck trouble, keep your chin slightly in and do not bend your neck back to its full extent. Hold this position for as long as is comfortable, breathing normally. Then return to an upright position and drop your arms.*

Triangle *Inhaling, raise your arms to the horizontal, and place your legs 60-90cm (24–36in) apart, pointing your right foot outward. Exhaling, bend to the right, without leaning forward, and slide your right hand down your leg toward your foot. Simultaneously, raise your left arm up, palm facing forward. Look up at your left hand. Hold the position, stretching up a little farther with each exhalation. Then, return to the starting position as you inhale. Repeat, bending to the left. Do not allow your hips to go backward as you bend to the side.*

PRONE ASANAS

These asanas flex your spine, stretch your abdomen, and tone your back muscles.

CAUTION ○ Avoid:

Prone Asanas for venous blood clots
Cobra for hernia, hypertension
Locust for hernia, hypertension, heart disease, low back pain
Bow for hernia, hypertension, heart disease, low back pain

Cobra Lie face down with your legs together. Place your hands flat on the floor, on either side of your chest. Inhaling, raise your head. Exhale. Inhaling, raise your chest until your ribs are off the floor. Exhale. Inhale and reach farther up and back, stopping just before your navel comes off the floor. Use your back muscles to lift your rib cage, and then use your arms. Hold for three to five breaths, then slowly "uncoil" as you exhale.

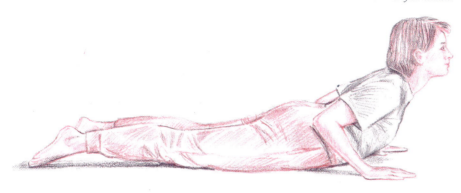

Locust Lie face down, with your legs together. Clench your fists, thumbs inside, and place them under your groin. Inhale and hold the breath, raising your right leg up straight, as far as is comfortable. Use only the leg and back muscles, keeping your upper body relaxed. Hold for three to ten breaths, then, slowly lower your leg as you exhale. Repeat for your left. Then, if you can, raise both legs together, following the same instructions as above.

Bow *Lie face down with your feet together. Then, bend your knees and bring your feet toward your head. Reach down with your hands and grasp your ankles. Then, as you inhale, pull on your feet to raise your thighs, chest, and head off the floor. Raise your upper and lower body as much as you comfortably can and rest on your abdomen. Keep your elbows straight. Initially your legs can be apart but bring them together as you gain proficiency. Feel the arch all along your back, like a drawn bow. Hold for at least three, and at most ten, breaths and release your legs as you exhale.*

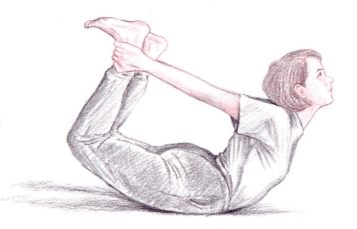

Crocodile *This is a relaxation posture, complementary to the Corpse (p. 37). Like a crocodile in the sun, lie face downward with your legs 30–60cm (12–24in) apart and your feet facing outward. Cradle your head in your arms or raise it on to your hands and elbows. With your eyes closed and your face relaxed, breathe from your abdomen, feeling it swell up and press down on the floor as you inhale and collapse as you exhale.*

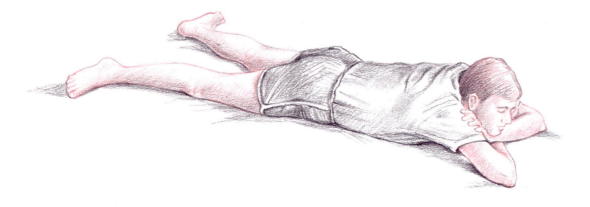

SUPINE ASANAS

These postures are effective, but they can be dangerous if you are unprepared. Master the *Half Shoulderstand* before you attempt the rest and make sure you are properly warmed up beforehand.

CAUTION ○ Avoid:

Supine Asanas for venous blood clots, heart disease, hypertension.
Half Shoulderstand for glaucoma, pressure in head and neck, obesity, fluid retention, menstruation.
Shoulderstand for glaucoma, pressure in head and neck, obesity, fluid retention, menstruation, neck pain, disc problems, weak back, painful breasts.
Plough for neck pain, obesity, disc problems, weak back, painful breasts.
Fish for neck pain, hyperactive thyroid.

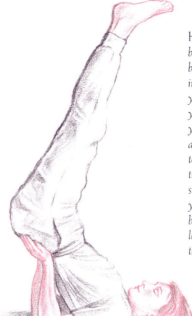

Half Shoulderstand *Lie on your back and raise your legs as you inhale, bending your knees if necessary. Exhaling, bring your legs farther back so your hips come off the floor. Support your hips with your hands, resting your weight on your arms, shoulders, and elbows. Inhaling, lift your legs up to the vertical position, but let your trunk remain at an angle of 45°. If the strain on your hands is too great, lower your legs toward your head. Hold, breathing normally, then bend your legs, release your arms, and roll out of the pose as you exhale.*

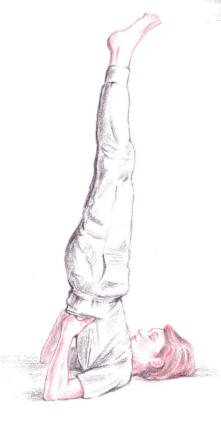

Shoulderstand *Start as if doing the Half Shoulderstand. When you have reached the full position, however, instead of letting your trunk remain at an angle, continue pushing upward until it is vertical. At the same time, slide your hands down toward your shoulders, wrapping your thumbs around the front and your fingers around the back. In the final position, your weight should be on your shoulders, not on your neck and head. Start by holding for half a minute and slowly increase this time to that recommended in the chart (p. 19). Breathe quietly and let your body relax. Come out as for the Half Shoulderstand.*

31

Plough *Start as you did for the Half Shoulderstand but instead of raising your legs to the vertical, stretch back and try to touch the ground behind you with your feet. You can also go direct from the Shoulderstand into the Plough by lowering your legs while supporting your waist with your hands. Release your arms as you do this, so they are stretched out flat, or fold them around your head. Hold, then roll out of the pose. If you can't get your legs down all the way, support your trunk with your arms until you are more flexible.*

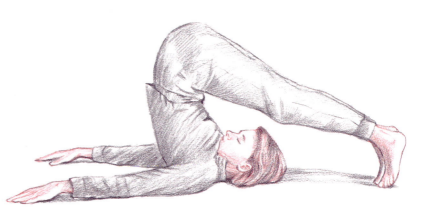

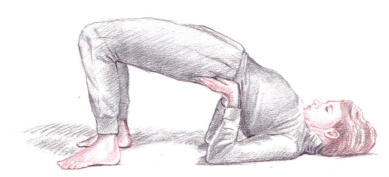

Bridge *Lie on your back, arms by your sides, with your knees bent and your legs slightly apart. As you inhale, push up with your feet and raise the mid part of your body as high as you comfortably can. Put your hands under your waist to support yourself. Feel the stretch along your thighs and abdomen. Relax your shoulders, neck, and face and breathe quietly. Hold this pose and then, to come out, gently lower your body to its original position as you exhale and straighten your legs.*

Fish *Sit with your legs outstretched and, exhaling, bend back slowly until your head touches the ground, supporting yourself on your elbows. Using your arms as levers, arch your back and neck up as far as you can. Be careful to take the weight on your arms and don't bend your head back too far, especially if you have neck problems. Hold for a third of the time you spent in the Shoulderstand. To come out of this pose, push up with your elbows to release your head and neck and slowly raise your upper body.*

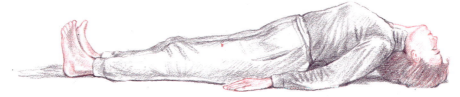

SITTING ASANAS

This cycle is calming and prepares you for *Relaxation* and *Pranayama*.

CAUTION ○ Avoid:

Sitting Asanas for venous blood clots, hyperacidity.
Moon for hypertension.
Camel for hernia, neck or back trouble.
Spinal Twist for disc problems, abdominal hernia or inflammation.
Forward Stretch for acute low back pain.

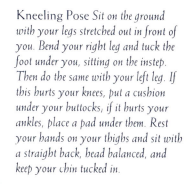

Kneeling Pose *Sit on the ground with your legs stretched out in front of you. Bend your right leg and tuck the foot under you, sitting on the instep. Then do the same with your left leg. If this hurts your knees, put a cushion under your buttocks; if it hurts your ankles, place a pad under them. Rest your hands on your thighs and sit with a straight back, head balanced, and keep your chin tucked in.*

Moon *Sit in the Kneeling Pose and grasp your right wrist behind your back. Exhaling, bend forward slowly from the waist until your forehead is on the ground. Hold this position, or rest your head on your knees if you find this difficult. Then, inhaling, slowly lift yourself back to the Kneeling Pose. Observe the changes in blood pressure in your head as you move your body up and down.*

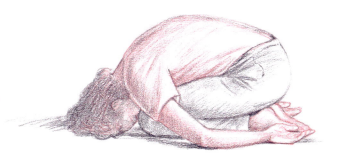

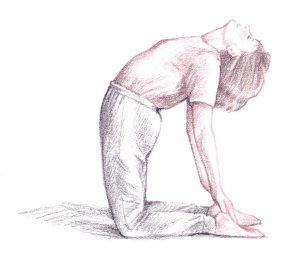

Camel *Kneel, but don't sit back on your heels. Inhaling, bend back, twisting to the right, and place your right hand on your right heel. Then, turn and place your left hand on your left heel. Arch forward, bringing your head and shoulders back. Breathe evenly for two minutes. Then, relax your arch and exhaling come up from the right side or sit back onto your heels. If you cannot reach your feet, start with your feet up on your toes, or only reach back to one side at a time.*

33

Spinal Twist *Sit with your legs stretched out in front of you. Raise your right leg and place your foot to the left of your other knee. Exhaling, turn to the right. Bring your left arm over and to the right of your upright knee, and grasp your shin, if you can. Gradually work farther down the leg until you can grasp your ankle. Rest your right hand on the floor behind you and keep your back straight. Each time you exhale twist a little farther right, using your arms to aid you, but do not force. After a few breaths relax and don't try to twist farther. Hold, then, release and repeat on the left.*

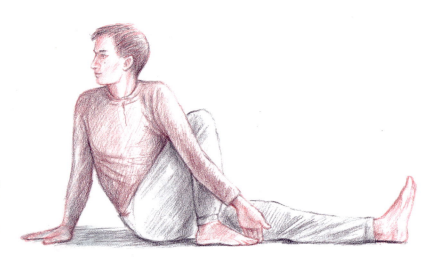

Forward Stretch *Sit with your legs straight in front of you and raise your arms above your head, palms facing forward. Stretch your body up from the bottom of the spine. Inhale, and bend forward as you exhale, reaching toward your toes. Bend from the hips, keeping your back as straight as you can. Each time you exhale, relax a little further. Pull in your abdomen and feel the stretch in your hamstrings. Hold the position, but do not strain, and avoid any sharp or acute pain.*

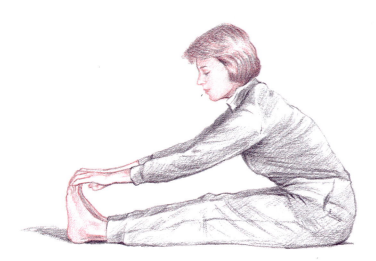

Supine Kneebend *Kneel, then take your feet out from under you, so they are next to your buttocks with your calves almost parallel to your thighs. Inhaling, lean back, supporting yourself on your elbows. Then, lie flat with your knees touching the ground, and rest your head on your folded arms. If you can't do this keep your legs under you and only come part of the way down. Hold, then slowly sit up.*

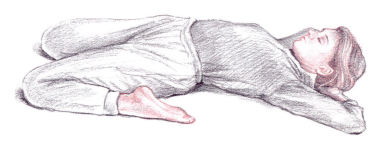

34

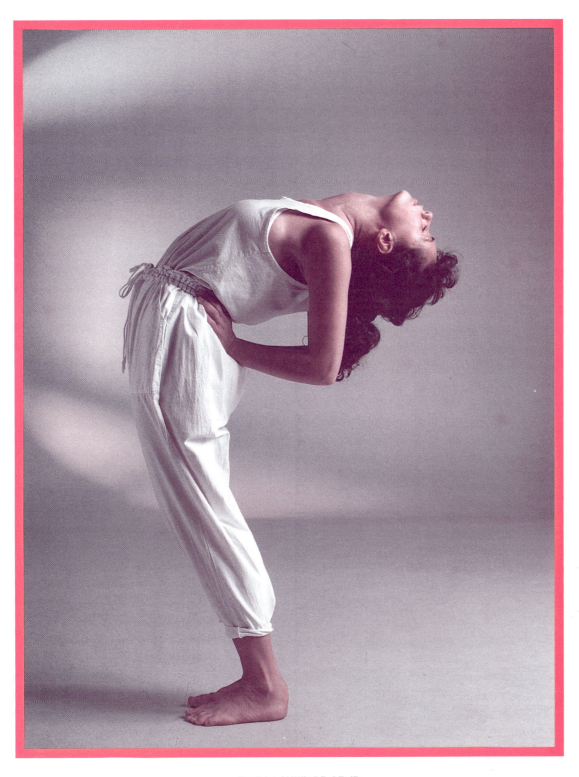

THE BACKWARD BEND

RELAXATION

There are three relaxation techniques given in this book: *Instant Relaxation Technique (IRT)* on page 23 takes two minutes; *Quick Relaxation Technique (QRT)*, opposite, takes five minutes; *Deep Relaxation Technique (DRT)*, opposite, takes between 10 and 20 minutes. Practise *IRT* after individual exercises and either *QRT* or *DRT* after the *Asanas*. You can also use any one on its own, to give rest during the day. Do both *DRT* and *QRT* while in the *Corpse* pose below, not the *IRT* version. Always come out of relaxation slowly.

THE CORPSE POSE

Lie on a firm, flat surface. Reduce the gap beneath your lower back by lifting your knees to your chest on your back, then slide your feet along the floor as you lower your legs. Spread your feet 20–30cm (8–12in) apart. Spread your arms so that they are 45cm (18in) from your body, palms upward. Lift your head and lower it with your chin tucked in. If this is uncomfortable, put a cushion under your head or rest your head on its side. Close your eyes and start either *QRT* or *DRT*.

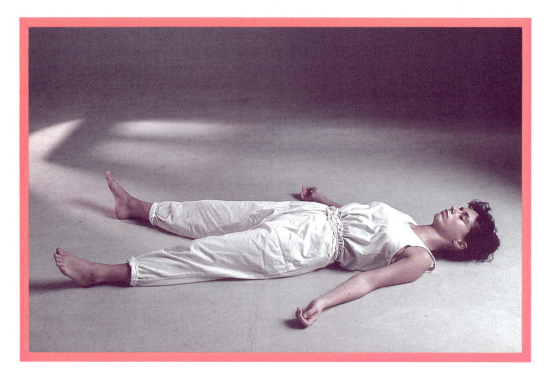

THE CORPSE

QUICK RELAXATION TECHNIQUE (QRT)

Be aware of your body lying on the floor. Note how your abdomen rises and falls as you breathe. Count ten cycles, noting how the movement becomes regular and slow as you observe it. For the next ten, feel your breath going into your abdomen as you inhale, expanding it like a balloon, then feel it collapse as you exhale. Do not breathe forcefully.

Next, feel yourself relax as you exhale and become energized by the incoming air as you inhale. Feel your body sink into the ground as your abdomen falls and the small pause before it rises again. As you inhale fully, feel your body become light and energetic. Enjoy the deep relaxation of exhaling and strengthen the energization of inhaling. Repeat ten times.

DEEP RELAXATION TECHNIQUE (DRT)

As you lie in the *Corpse* pose, follow the instructions below. At first it may be easier to record them on a cassette and play it back to yourself. Read them slowly and pause for several seconds after each instruction. Later, you will be able to practise without such aids and relaxation will become spontaneous. This sequence is also used in *Yoga Nidra* on page 59.

Either dictate or learn the following: "Close your eyes and relax your body stage by stage, beginning from the toes ... Feel a tingling in the tips of your toes and the roots of your toenails ... Relax your toes ... the soles of your feet ... your ankles ... all of your feet ... Relax your calf muscles ... your knees ... your thighs ... your buttocks ... Relax all of your legs from your toes to your buttocks ... inhale deeply and chant 'AH', feeling the vibrations in your abdomen travel down to your toes ... Be aware of your abdomen and thorax ... Feel the surge of energy each time you inhale and your upper body expands ... Feel the waves of relaxation as you exhale travel outward ... Feel a tingling in the tips of your fingers and the roots of your fingernails ... Relax the muscles of your hands, arms, waist, back, and shoulders ... Loosen your spine, vertebra by vertebra ... Be aware of your chest ... Inhale and chant 'OO', feeling the vibrations in your chest cavity spread down to your arms and fingers ... Relax your throat and then face... Start with your chin ... Now your lower jaw ... your teeth ... the root of your tongue ... Now your palate and upper jaw ... your cheeks and cheek bones ... Relax your lips, keeping a beautiful smile on your face ... Relax your nose ... the space between your eyebrows ... eyes ... forehead ... ears ... scalp ... back of the head ... Inhale deeply and hum 'MM', feeling the vibration in your throat spread through your head ... Now relax your entire body ... relax ... totally relax ... Inhale and chant 'OM' ... feel the vibrations from your toes to your head ... Imagine a vast ocean or sky ... merge with the ocean or sky ... Dive deeper and deeper into the ocean of silence."

PRANAYAMA

Yogic breathing, or *Pranayama*, is central to the daily session. Just as the *Asanas* that precede it slow down the physical body, the breathing exercises shown here harmonize the flow of *prana* within you (pp. 10–11).

There are three different types of breathing: abdominal, thoracic, and clavicular. In natural breathing we use all three types at once, so all the muscles involved are exercised. But when we breathe badly one of the three types of breathing tends to be underused and the muscles that bring it about become weak or chronically tense. The exercises that follow relax and strengthen these breathing muscles and also teach you how to use the three types of breathing in a balanced way. Sit in the *Kneeling Pose* (p. 33), or any other comfortable position, with your back straight. Always breathe slowly and evenly, unless instructed otherwise, and stop for a moment after inhaling or exhaling. Be as relaxed as possible, let your body breathe by itself, and just guide it with the minimum of effort.

CAUTION Avoid *Rapid Abdominal Breathing* for hypertension or epilepsy, during menstruation, and read page 17 if you have had abdominal surgery.

Sectional Breathing *Inhale by letting your abdomen bulge and then, exhale by drawing it in continuously and slowly. While learning, place one of your hands on your abdomen. Keep your chest and shoulders stationary. Next, hold your shoulders and abdomen still as you inhale by expanding your rib cage. Exhale by slowly releasing your ribs. While learning, place your palms on the sides of your chest to feel the movement and push gently inward in the last stage of the exhalation. Then, hold your abdomen slightly in, rib cage stationary, and breathe in and out by allowing your shoulders to move up and down. Finally combine all three, inhaling from your abdomen, continuing with the ribs, and ending the breath with the clavicles. Exhale in the reverse order.*

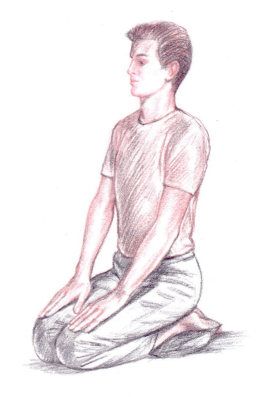

RAPID ABDOMINAL BREATHING

Keeping your neck, shoulders, and face relaxed, exhale forcibly using your abdomen, and then inhale passively by relaxing it. Repeat, letting your abdomen go in and out rhythmically. Begin by doing three rounds of ten breaths. Add ten breaths each week until you reach 30 per round. Relax for 20 seconds between rounds, slowing or stopping your breathing. Start with one breath every two seconds, gradually speeding up to two breaths every second. Make sure you have mastered the movement before you increase the number of breaths.

Alternate-nostril Breathing Tuck the first and second fingers of your right hand into your palm, extending your thumb and the fourth and fifth fingers. Close the right nostril with your thumb. Exhale and inhale through the left nostril. Then, close your left nostril with the fourth and fifth fingers and open your right; exhale and inhale through the right nostril. Repeat the cycle at least five times. Keep your breathing slow, even, deep, and silent. Try to follow the course of the breath down the nose and throat into the lungs, and then out again.

Folded-tongue Breathing Fold your tongue back and place its tip against the root of your upper front teeth. Inhale slowly and evenly, around each side of your tongue, and note the cold air come into your mouth and travel down your throat. Exhale through your nose.

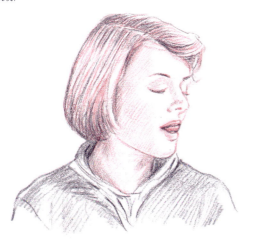

SOUNDS BREATHING

Inhale deeply and then, loudly vocalize the sound "AH" as you exhale. Imagine that the vibration permeates your abdomen and spreads down your legs to your toes. Repeat three times. Now repeat, but vocalize the sound "OO" and let the vibration in your chest spread down your arms to your fingers. Next, use "MM", a humming sound made with closed lips. The vibration starts in your throat and extends to your face and head. End by chanting "OM", three times, and feeling the vibration throughout your body.

39

MEDITATION

Meditation is the heart of yoga. It is the flowering of the mind and soul, and with it comes peace, clarity, harmony, and energy.

Choose a word, such as "OM" or "GOD" or "ONE", and chant it inwardly to yourself. Do not move your lips, just hear the sound in your mind. At first repeat it over and over, several times during each breath, and let your thoughts come and pass away without becoming involved with them. When you establish a rhythm, slow down the chanting but speed up if disturbing thoughts interfere and only slow down again when a rhythm is restored.

When you have mastered this, make the internal sound loudly and deeply and feel an imaginary vibration from it throughout your body. Let the word start quietly, swell to a loud, vibrating sound, and then fade away into silence. Gradually lengthen the sound over more than one breathing cycle. Then, let it become continuous, swelling and dwindling like a gentle wave. Finally, let it fade away and dwell in the silence. Observe your thoughts rising and falling, without becoming involved in them, but if you become caught up in them resume the chanting. Finish by sending out good thoughts to those near you, those you know, and all other living beings.

Practise meditation after *Pranayama*. The full practice takes 15 minutes, but five minutes regularly will provide substantial benefits.

Meditation Pose *Sit with your legs out straight and part them to form a V shape. Bend your right leg and bring it toward you, placing your right foot on the floor close to your groin. Then bend your left leg and place your left foot on the floor close to your right leg. Rest your hands on your knees, as shown. Keep your back straight, and start to meditate. If you cannot hold the pose for the time necessary, try the* Kneeling Pose *(p. 33) or sit in a chair.*

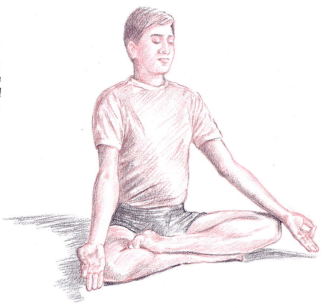

EMOTION CULTURING

There were once three starving beggars. The first beggar had his bowl filled, but the second and third had only half a bowl each. The second beggar ate his portion full of resentment that he had less than the first; the third was just grateful to have some food and thoroughly enjoyed it. In the same way, it is for you to choose whether to see the positive or the negative side of things – whether to regard your bowl as half empty or half full.

It is all too easy to fall into negative states of thinking, with feelings of anger, resentment, hate, inferiority, and ruthless personal ambition governing your actions and life. These take their toll on both your own health and that of others close to you, and rarely work to anyone's advantage. *Emotion Culturing* can help you to transform such negative states into positive ones.

Two techniques are used to bring this change about. The first is *intensive* and involves consciously evoking positive emotions and amplifying them, while at the same time diffusing negative states of mind. You can do this in *Yoga Nidra* (p. 59) or by singing, chanting, or dancing. These have been used by both traditional religions and modern psychotherapy to cultivate positive states of mind.

In your day-to-day transactions you can utilize *extensive* techniques. Here you take one of your more extreme emotions, such as anger or panic, and decide to avoid feeling this way for a few months. Then every night, before you go to bed, recall the events of the day and write down any lapses you might have had. The next morning strengthen your resolution. Initially you will have many lapses but soon you will become aware of when the negative emotion is swelling within you. This will help you reduce its intensity and maybe even to avoid it altogether.

Use these techniques to diffuse violent, self-destructive emotions and replace them with feelings of love, caring, understanding, and happiness. Then negative feelings will cease to dominate you; you will become emotionally steady and balanced and able to handle the most demanding situations with equanimity and poise.

RECOLLECTION AND DWELLING IN SILENCE
Try to hold the peace you experienced during meditation, recollecting it at times during the day. When faced with a challenging situation, return to that peace momentarily if you can. This helps you stand back from your problems and gives you perspective. And when you have a few moments to spare, try "dwelling in silence" rather than further occupying your mind.

Diet and Lifestyle

To succeed in your search for health and wellbeing you need to establish a diet and lifestyle that will sustain and promote a positive approach. The yogic diet, developed by yogis long ago as they strove for mastery over "the self", can be a tool for this. The yogis realized that diet has a profound effect on both the mind and body, and that you cannot attain true mastery over your mind without balance in your diet and lifestyle.

Using their highly developed internal awareness, yogis classified food into three categories: *tamasic*, or impure foods, which had a negative or harmful effect on the body and mind, and actually drained their resources; *rajasic*, or stimulating, which tended to raise levels of physical activity and led to emotional upsurges, but were detrimental in the long term; and *sattvic*, or pure, which were the most health-promoting, adding vitality and energy to the whole body in a balanced way.

In general, *tamasic* foods today are stale, tasteless, or actually spoiled and include those with a foul odour, those that contain artificial additives, and those that are overprocessed or produced by factory farming. They are also foods that lead to dependency, such as alcohol or coffee. These make you dull, lazy, drowsy, and unable to think clearly. *Rajasic* foods are spicy, excessively sour, bitter, pungent, or roasted. Concentrated sources of protein, such as meat, fish, and eggs are also *rajasic*. These make you physically active, but also make you more aggressive and restless. *Sattvic* foods are the purest, those that are fresh, fragrant, and tasty. They include organically grown natural foods, without additives, such as fresh vegetables and fruits, cereals, dairy products, nuts, and seeds. These help to maintain clarity of thought, decision-making, and intellectual and contemplative thinking. They also increase your vitality, energy, and health and make you more joyful, cheerful, and calm.

While practising yoga you should eat *sattvic* foods. Try to reduce the variety of foods you eat as well, and allow yourself to see that your happiness does not depend on eating many kinds of tasty foods. Mastering such cravings for food, without losing your poise and happiness in life, is a path of yoga comparable in importance to *Asanas*, *Pranayama*, and *Meditation*. The aim is to achieve moderation, which is the basis of a balanced diet in yoga, and remove overindulgence in any form of food.

Start gradually, cutting down not only the variety but also the quantity and frequency of food consumption. In the first few weeks of yoga have no snacks between meals and start reducing your consumption of stimulant drinks, such as tea, coffee, and soft drinks. Have only three meals a day (or even two). When you first start to do this, you may feel unpleasant symptoms such as headaches, nausea, or loss of concentration. This is because your body is clearing accumulated toxins from your tissues. Be careful not to eat too little. If you start to feel dizzy or faint, or even slightly tired and edgy, you may have hypoglycaemia. In this case, revert to your former diet until you have consulted a doctor. Hypoglycaemic people need to eat small amounts of food at frequent intervals to maintain their blood sugar levels during the day

The way you eat is also important and, in yoga, eating is regarded as a sacred act. Try to have your meals in a quiet, pleasant frame of mind, giving full attention to the food and allowing your body to turn over its resources to the task of digestion, which is disturbed if you are under stress or distracted. Do not read or watch TV while you eat; just chat or quietly enjoy the food. You will find that you utilize it more effectively, and many minor digestive problems will spontaneously clear up.

The same yogic principles as for diet apply to other aspects of daily life. The general aim is to establish a well-ordered, calm life. Make your surroundings clean and pleasant, yet simple, extending this principle to dress and other major elements of your environment. Seek to create a life that enhances awareness and sensitivity, both of yourself and of others.

Try and establish a set of "dos" and "don'ts", a code for living that you feel comfortable with, and avoid acting in ways that give rise to conflict within you. Yogis have a traditional set of "don'ts", or *yamas*. These include *ahimsa*, the principle of nonviolence made famous by Gandhi, but there are others such as avoiding untruth, excessive possessions, or overindulgence in sex. These principles may not suit you, but you can construct a code for yourself, based on your own ideals. Also try to promote positive actions that benefit yourself and others. Traditional yogic "dos", or *niyamas*, include cleanliness in all parts of life, maintaining enthusiasm and joy, perseverance, self-analysis and introspection, and love of God. Again, these may not be views that you feel you can share wholeheartedly. It is up to you to search within yourself to find what you want to do. Trying to raise your level of consciousness and its expression in actions is a challenge – but if you persevere you will soon begin to learn the art of self-responsibility and of living at peace with yourself and your environment.

Aim to broaden your horizons – try to develop tolerance, sensitivity, and compassion in your views and relationships. When the ability to live in peace, with yourself and others, becomes second nature your whole life will become joyful. This will create the right basis for the growing unity of humanity as we approach the 21st century.

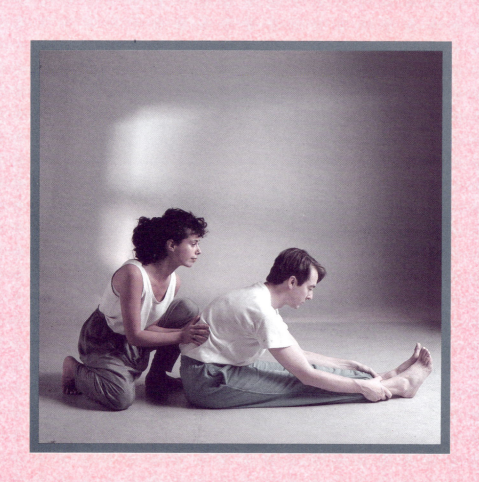

THE AILMENTS

Ailments can be either *functional* or *organic*. Functional ailments involve disturbances to your body systems and include minor stress-related disorders. These can often be completely cured by yoga. Organic ailments usually involve some form of physical damage; this may be curable, as with some infections, or incurable, as with a damaged heart. Most organic ailments, however, respond well to yoga practice, especially if they have a strong psychosomatic element.

Yoga can help you to manage such organic ailments on many levels, improving your quality of life and even increasing life expectancy. In the form of the *Basic Session* (pp. 16–43), yoga can often help to relieve the symptoms of illness and reduce your need for medication, bringing with it a great increase in your level of well being.

To treat specific ailments with yoga you must modify the daily *Basic Session* according to your needs. Certain yoga practices are particularly beneficial for certain ailments, while others must be avoided. To find out how to create a personal yoga session, designed for *you* and *your* needs, read fully the advice given for each of the ailments from which you suffer. At the end of each, where applicable, there is an advice box that tells you which practices to "emphasize" from the *Basic Session*, and which to "avoid". You may also find that some additional practices, illustrated in *The Ailments* section, are listed under "add". Using the information in the advice box, go back to pages 17–19 where the *Basic Session* is explained. Then, to create your own table of exercises, delete all the practices listed under "avoid" and insert any "add" practices in the appropriate positions. Give more time to these, and also to those in the "emphasize" list, always including them in your daily session. If you have more than one ailment, combine all the "avoids" for your ailments, deleting them from your session, and only do the exercises that remain in the table (p. 19) and any additional exercises.

As you become familiar with the daily session, expand your scope by reading other books and consulting experienced yoga practitioners at every opportunity. But seek advice when you modify your daily session, to make sure you are on the right path.

WHOLE BODY

In our fast-moving modern society we have eliminated many traditional diseases, only to find them replaced by the new affliction of stress. We often express mental tensions physically and stress plays an important part in the cause, maintenance, and aggravation of many ailments. It is becoming increasingly obvious that our physical health cannot be separated from our emotional and mental wellbeing.

Your muscles, joints, and ligaments are quite frequently affected. Stress is often reflected in spasm, a constant muscular contraction, which squanders your energy and leads to fatigue and either general or local body aches. Stress can also overstimulate your mind, causing insomnia and eating disorders, and attack your immune system, making you more susceptible to rheumatoid arthritis and other immune-related ailments.

Yoga can help you improve all these conditions and prevent them from becoming chronic ailments. If you suspect that you are overstressed, try the stress-management programme in this section (pp. 53-5), which is specially designed for those with a busy lifestyle.

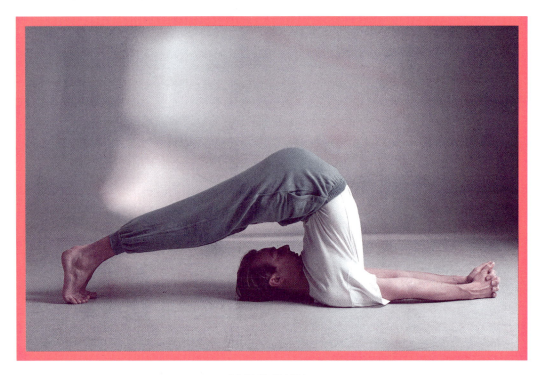

THE PLOUGH

BACK PAIN

Our upright stance is one of evolution's most remarkable achievements. The shape of our spine allows us to balance erect and our strong back muscles maintain the posture by partial contraction. This, however, makes them prone to spasm – a state of constant over-contraction that results in back pain.

Stress is one of the main causes, though injury too can induce "protective" spasm and delay the healing process. Where back pain is due to major damage, such as a slipped disc, inflammation, or infection, you will need the guidance of a yoga specialist to practise yoga safely. If it is due to stress or minor injury, yoga helps you to release the spasm by making you aware of tensions and relaxing you.

Start the *Basic Session* gradually, introducing side- and back-bending after two or more weeks, and forward bending after a month. If you suffer from severe pain, only work on the least painful parts of the back until you feel relaxed and mentally prepared. If you have neck pains avoid the *Shoulderstand, Plough* (p. 31), and *Fish* (p. 32). For lower back pain avoid all *Loosening Up* (pp. 22-3), except the *Embryo,* and the *Sun Salute* (pp. 24-5) and take care while bending forward. For disc problems avoid or minimize twisting.

After a few weeks, try diffusing the pain. When a stretch starts to be painful, imagine that at each exhalation you are radiating the pain into your surroundings. But take care and avoid any pain that is more than mild. Cultivate a caring awareness of your body.

FROM THE BASIC SESSION
● Emphasize: *Cat Stretch; Twisting; Embryo; Cobra; Locust; Spinal Twist; Alternate-nostril Breathing; Meditation; Emotion Culturing.*
FROM THE AILMENTS SECTION
⊕ Add: *Abdominal Lock (p. 74); Supine Twist (below).*

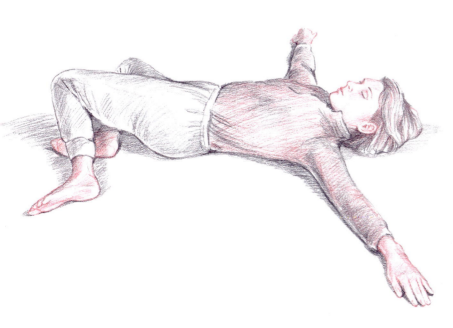

Supine Twist *Lie down and raise your knees, sliding your feet up to your buttocks. Stretch out your arms. Inhale, then, exhaling lower your knees to the floor on your right. If this is painful, only lower them part way. Inhaling, raise your knees up again then, exhaling, lower them to your left. Raise and lower them from side to side several times, in synchrony with your breathing. Then raise them up, exhale, and inhaling, stretch out your legs. Practise after* Single-leg Raising. CAUTION *Avoid* Supine Twist *during menstruation.*

RHEUMATISM AND ARTHRITIS

Joints, and the soft tissues that support them, are the most vulnerable areas of your skeletal frame. They act as shock absorbers for your bones, bearing the brunt of weight and exercise, yet they must also be flexible to allow free movement. As you get older, they tend to wear out and you may start to develop one of the numerous joint conditions generally known as rheumatism or arthritis.

These ailments can be divided into three basic groups: those that are strongly stress related, such as fibromyalgia and rheumatoid arthritis; those that are partly due to the ageing process, such as osteoarthrosis, and generalized joint aches and pains; and others, such as ankylosing spondylitis (commonly known as bamboo-spine disease).

If you suffer from a stress-linked rheumatic ailment, the three-layered approach of yoga therapy – relaxing your muscles, slowing your breathing, and calming your mind – can bring you great benefits. Rheumatoid arthritis, for example, can respond particularly well to yoga therapy. It is due to an autoimmune conflict that affects both muscles and joints, causing pain, chronic fatigue, and inflammation. Here, yoga meditation balances your immune system and stretching exercises release your stiff joints. The cleansing effect of yoga also increases the effectiveness of anti-inflammatory drugs, helping you to reduce your dosage.

In fibromyalgia, which can last three or more years, the supporting tissues and muscles close to certain joints become tender and ache and this is often followed by uneasy sleep and depression. Early research on the effects of yoga therapy has yielded promising results, but suggests that regular practice over several months is needed to improve this difficult condition appreciably.

Ageing-related joint conditions are also aggravated by stress but are primarily caused by chronic ill use of the joints. Long-term inactivity makes the joints stiff and painful, as in osteoarthrosis, and overuse, for example in athletes, strains the joints and makes them wear out more quickly. Yoga can help you by stimulating blood circulation, removing accumulated wastes, and releasing stiffened joints.

Osteoarthrosis mainly affects load-bearing joints, such as the knees, hips, and spine. If you often have knee pains, practise *Single-leg Raising* (p. 21), and for hip pain practise the *Embryo* (p. 23). Generalized joint pains, or arthralgias, tend to affect the whole body. Here, relaxation, meditation, and gradual, passive loosening of the joints is the most effective treatment.

In ankylosing spondylitis, a hereditary inflammatory disease, the vertebrae in the spine fuse together, making it rigid and causing pain. Yogic exercises that flex the spine free these immobile joints and reduce the stiffening. Even if you experience some lumbar pain, you need not avoid forward bending. Do not strain, however, and avoid excessive pain.

For all types of joint disorder practise the *Basic Session* slowly and cautiously, without straining or overstretching. *Never* move actively inflamed joints. Try to relax into the *Asanas* gently and avoid acute pain. Concentrate on the *Passive Loosening* exercises on pages 49-51 to mobilize stiff joints and cultivate yogic attitudes in everyday life (p. 41).

FROM THE BASIC SESSION
● Emphasize: *Rapid Abdominal Breathing; Meditation; Emotion Culturing.*
FROM THE AILMENTS SECTION
⊕ Add: *Passive Loosening (pp. 49-51)*

PASSIVE LOOSENING

Tension in the neck and the shoulders can cause bad posture, headaches, frozen shoulder, pain, and joint problems. Neck exercises (below) release this tension, and the exercises on pages 50-1 flex the joints. Sit erect, keep your eyes closed, and shoulders relaxed. Practise instead of *Loosening Up*.

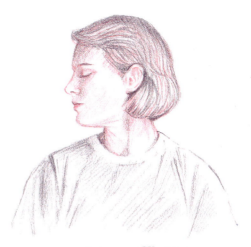

Side-to-side Rotation *Keeping your chin in, very slowly and evenly turn your head to the left – as far as it will comfortably go. Hold for a few moments, then, turn to the right. Hold for a few moments, then, face front. This cycle should take about one to two minutes. Repeat three times and go on to Forward-backward Flexing.*

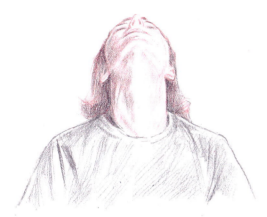

Forward-backward Flexing *Face front, then, tilt your head forward so your chin comes in toward your sternum. Then, tilt backward slowly, keeping your chin in. Bring the head back up to the starting position. Repeat five times, giving each cycle about five seconds. Now go on to* Circling and Shoulder-lifting.

Circling and Shoulder-lifting *Tilt your head forward and roll it to the right, so your right ear is close to your shoulder. Then, raise it upright and lean over to the left, bringing your left ear near your left shoulder. Roll your head to the front, the initial position, thus completing a full circle. Do this five times clockwise and five times counterclockwise. Next, raise each shoulder five times, then, both together five times. Move on to pages 50-1.*

49

1 Clenching Your Fist *Sit in a comfortable position, with your back straight, and hold your right wrist with your left hand. Clench your right hand into a fist, with your thumb inside your fingers, then, open it again. Repeat five times, and then, switch hands and do the same thing with your left. Move on to exercise 2.*

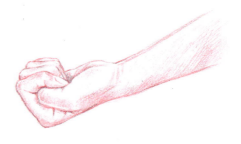

2 Circling Your Wrist *Support your right arm with your left hand. Make a loose fist with your right hand, folding the thumb between the fingers, and rotate it in a clockwise direction several times. Then, do the same counterclockwise. Change hands and rotate your left wrist as above. Finish by rotating both wrists simultaneously, holding your unsupported arms before you. Move on to exercise 3.*

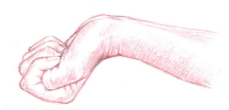

3 Hand Up and Down *Sit in the same position as above, holding your right forearm with your left hand. Extend the fingers of your right hand out straight, or as straight as you can manage. Move your hand up and down several times, flexing at the wrist, holding your fingers and palm straight. Then change hands and repeat for your left. Now move on to exercise 4.*

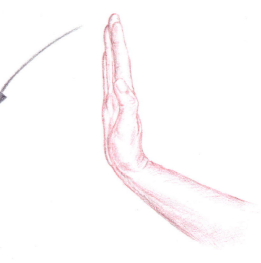

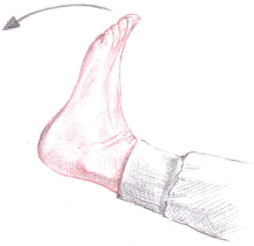

4 Flexing Your Toes *Sit in a chair and raise your right leg, supporting it with your hands (see position 6). Move your toes and foot up and down, flexing your ankle joint. Stretch your toes toward you as they come up and away from you as they go down. Repeat with your other leg. Go on to exercise 5 when you have finished.*

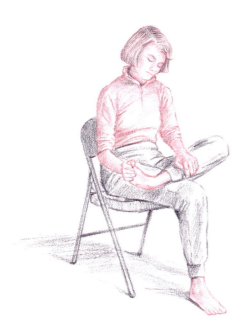

5 Stretching Your Ankle *Sit in the chair as shown and rest your right leg on your left thigh. Support your right leg with your right hand and use the other hand to rotate your foot passively. Rotate it five times in a clockwise direction and five times in a counterclockwise direction. Let your foot remain relaxed while you do this. Then change legs and repeat on the other side. Move on to exercise 6.*

6 Flexing Your Knees *Sit in the chair as shown and support your right leg with your hands. Raise your lower leg from the knee until your whole leg is straight, then, lower it again. Repeat several times. Switch legs and repeat as above. Now move on to exercise 7.*

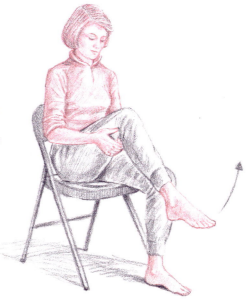

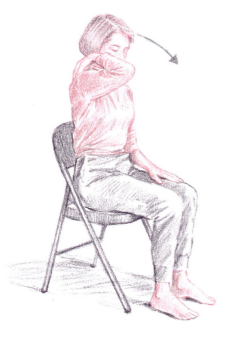

7 Stretching Your Elbows *Sit in a chair as shown. Raise your right arm in front of you, keeping it horizontal and in line with your shoulder. Bend your arm at the elbow and reach back to touch your shoulder with your right hand. Then extend it again, so your arm is straight. Do not move your upper arm while you do this. Repeat several times, then, do the same with your left arm.*

51

ABDOMINAL HERNIA

The abdomen contains many vital organs that keep you alive and well and that are confined and protected by the muscles in the abdomen. A hernia occurs when these muscles are weakened and a gap is made in the abdominal wall from which part of an internal organ bulges out.

Such weakness can either be congenital or else caused by surgery or lack of exercise. After surgery the suture lines are vulnerable sites, while insufficient exercise weakens your muscles and burdens your abdomen with excess fat. Straining these weakened muscles by lifting heavy weights or even through chronic coughing or constipation, can create a gap and result in a hernia.

Yoga cannot cure this. Once a gap has been made, hernia-repair surgery is necessary to close it. It can help you avoid a recurrence, however, by strengthening your abdominal muscles, reducing fat, and promoting body awareness. It can also help to prevent a hernia occurring after abdominal surgery.

You must wait at least two weeks before starting yoga if you have undergone hernia-repair surgery; longer if you have had other major surgery. Then start yoga gradually, under the supervision of your doctor or a yoga specialist. Practise *Single-leg Raising* (p. 23) three times a day, but only raise your legs up to 60° and work up to 20 raises for each leg. Avoid any strain to your abdomen.

CAUTION Consult your doctor before starting yoga if you have undergone any form of abdominal surgery.

FROM THE BASIC SESSION
● Emphasize: *Embryo; Half Shoulderstand; Sectional Breathing; Rapid Abdominal Breathing.*
○ Avoid: *Double-leg Raising; Jogging; Forward-backward Bending; Sideways Bending; Twisting; Sun Salute; Prone Asanas; Camel.*
FROM THE AILMENTS SECTION
⊕ Add: *Head-lifting (below); Abdominal Lock (p. 74); Abdominal Pumping (p. 76).*

Head-lifting *Lie down, with your legs out straight and your arms by your sides. Exhale and raise your head, shoulders, and arms. Hold for a moment, and then, inhale, come down and relax. Repeat up to 20 times. Avoid this exercise if you feel pain in your abdomen or neck; or only come up part way at first, and work up to the full position gradually. Insert after Single-leg Raising.*

JETLAG

Long-distance air travel makes many demands on your system. When you move across time zones your physiological clock has to "reset" its 24-hour cycle – and you also have to cope with deadlines, delays, and unfamiliar situations. There are noise, bustle, and changes in pressure, climate, and culture. You can, however, greatly reduce these additional stresses through simple yogic practices.

While travelling, take note of feelings of tension and fatigue as they arise and don't escape by drinking alcohol, smoking, or trying to become absorbed in a novel or film.

Simple awareness will by itself reduce your stress level but you can reduce it further by slowing your breathing and (when possible) by *QRT* (p. 37) and *Meditation* (p. 40). Also, try to imagine that you have been living at your destination's time for 24 hours already to help your mind "reset" its internal clock.

When you have arrived at your destination, allow at least 24 hours before you become active. Take a walk, or practise yoga before you sleep. If you are very tired, start with *Cyclic Meditation* (pp. 54-5) and go on to the *Basic Session* as your energies return.

STRESS

The stress reaction is a natural response to fear or uncertainty. When you feel anxious, afraid, or upset, it prepares your body to fight or flee from danger. Most stress-inducing experiences we face today, however, can't be resolved either by fighting or by flight, or by any direct physical action, so stress remains unexpressed and unrelieved.

Chronic stress is the major challenge of the technological era. Stresses can pile up without your noticing, each tension feeding others, until you become chronically overstimulated. Eventually, this is expressed as physical disease or mental disorders.

Yoga helps you break this vicious circle by teaching you to slow down and diffuse stress. Many nonyogic relaxation techniques fail to do this, because the process is blocked by a lack of awareness. Every relaxation tends to be followed by a stagnation, at which point the

mind becomes active and prevents you relaxing further. *Cyclic Meditation* (pp. 54-5), overcomes this by alternating relaxation with a physical stimulation that occupies and stills your mind, allowing you to relax more deeply.

Practise *Cyclic Meditation* every day and the *Short Basic Session*, when you have the time. The *Instant Relaxation Technique* (IRT - p. 23) and *Quick Relaxation Technique* (QRT - p. 37) can also be used on their own to cut the spiral of developing tensions at work. If you don't have time for the full *Cyclic Meditation* sequence, you can omit either the standing or sitting postures, alternating them from day to day.

These exercises, and cultivating yogic attitudes in everyday life (p. 41), will help you to relax and to face the most testing situations without getting worked up. Your way of life itself will become more holistic, characterized by calmness, peace, poise, and efficiency.

53

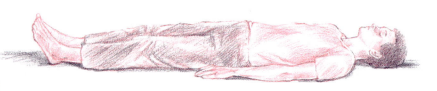

CYCLIC MEDITATION

The exercises in *Cyclic Meditation* are all taken from the *Basic Session*, but are done in a special order and with a different mental state. *Cyclic Meditation* can either replace or be done in addition to the *Basic Session*, or be used as a form of meditation – but go more slowly for this and extend DRT to 20 minutes. Practise in a quiet room, ideally in the evening before you eat. Wait 30 minutes after a snack and 90 minutes after a full meal. Never alter the order of the exercises and keep your eyes closed throughout the sequence.

1 Instant Relaxation Technique (IRT) *Lie as above, with your legs together and arms by your side. Tense all your muscles then relax as in Basic Session IRT (p. 23). The whole exercise should take about two minutes. Then, turn onto your left side and note the effect of this changed position on your body. Slowly stand up, keeping your eyes closed, and go on to the Lateral Arc.*

2 Lateral Arc *Stand up straight, always keeping your eyes closed. Then, perform the Lateral Arc (p. 27) very slowly. Observe the stretch along your outer side, and the compression and touch of your palm on the inner side where it touches the leg. Notice how the blood comes into your hand as you lower it, the after effects of the stretch, and any changes in your breathing. Go on to the Hands-to-feet Pose.*

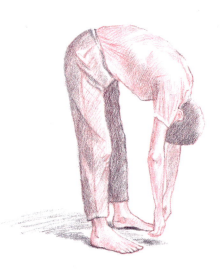

3 Hands-to-feet Pose *Slowly bend forward to the Hands-to-feet Pose (p. 27). Maintain your awareness of the various sensations in your body as you do this: note the rise in blood pressure to your head and the stretch along the back of your legs. Remain in this position for at least two minutes, relaxing, then return slowly, noting the lightness in your head as you come up. Wait for a while until this passes and go on to the Backward Bend.*

54

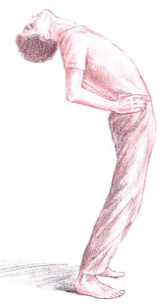

4 Backward Bend *Again, stand up straight, then lean back into the Backward Bend (p. 28). Maintain this position for about two minutes, unless you start to feel dizzy or uncomfortable. Note the stretch all along the front of your body. Come out of the posture slowly, noting the flood of nerve impulses as you release the stretch and come up. Keep your eyes closed and lower yourself to the floor carefully and do the Quick Relaxation Technique (QRT).*

5 Quick Relaxation Technique (QRT) *First lie on your right side for a few seconds; observe the sensations in your body. Then assume the classical Corpse Pose, shown on page 36, with your arms and legs slightly spread out. Practise the Quick Relaxation Technique on page 37; observe the deepening relaxation and the energy surge that you feel as your lungs fill with oxygen. The whole of this sequence should last for three or four minutes. Now move on to the Moon.*

6 Moon *Sit up, without turning on to your side, using your arms to help you. Sit with your legs straight out in front and put your arms behind you, keeping them straight, too. Hold this position for about 30 seconds. Then, assume the Kneeling Pose (p. 38) and hold for another 30 seconds. Slowly lower yourself down into the Moon (p. 33), noting the increased blood pressure to your head. Hold this for about two minutes, return to the Kneeling Pose, and from there go into the Camel.*

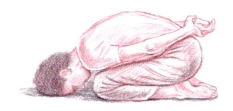

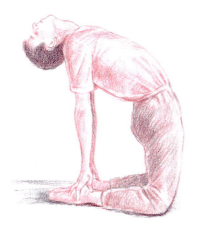

7 Camel *From kneeling, go into the Camel (p. 33) or the Half Camel (also p. 33). Hold for two minutes, being aware of the stretch, then return to the Kneeling Pose. Note the stimuli that result from the stretch. Then go into the Corpse pose (p. 36) and perform Deep Relaxation Technique (DRT – p. 37), for at least ten minutes. When you finish, come up straight, without using your arms. Assume a comfortable position, and open your eyes in your own time. Try to maintain the relaxed state throughout the rest of the day.*

55

FATIGUE

Chronic fatigue, induced and maintained by stress, is a common feature of modern life. Unlike the fatigue created by intense physical work, from which you soon recover with a good rest, chronic fatigue is generalized and ordinary forms of rest bring little respite. Mental tensions are often expressed as constant partial contraction of your muscles, which depletes your energy and disrupts your breathing pattern, making you continuously tired. Your muscles remain tense even when you are inactive and resting, so until you reduce your stress levels you cannot get relief.

To combat fatigue, start the day with the *Short Basic Session* (p. 19), emphasizing the *Asanas* (pp. 26-35) and *DRT* (p. 37). But take care not to exhaust yourself. In the evening, restore your depleted energy levels by practising *DRT*, *Pranayama* (pp. 38-9), and *Meditation* (p. 40) for 20 to 30 minutes. If you feel tired during the day, relax in the *Inverted Corpse* (p. 62) for a few minutes.

Excessive, sudden, or unexplained fatigue can also be caused by major illnesses. Though yoga may be able to help, you should first consult your doctor for a diagnosis.

INSOMNIA

You need to sleep a certain amount every day in order to feel truly well. Sleep is essential, as it gives your mind and body a chance to rest and recuperate by withdrawing from action. Many people though, can only sleep by using sleeping pills or tranquillizers. Despite being addictive and possibly harmful, these are the most frequently used drugs in the world.

Yoga can provide a natural solution to the problem of long-term sleeplessness. Insomnia is usually caused by excessive tension and anxiety, which stops the brain from "switching off" at night. When you get into bed, all the unfinished mental tasks and unexpressed tensions surface – thoughts and emotions spin around your mind and produce a constant internal stimulation that keeps you tense. Instead of using pills, however, you can use simple yogic techniques to calm anxiety and slow down the mind.

Before getting into bed do *Arm-stretch Breathing* ten times and *Hand-stretch Breathing* six times. Once in bed spend a few minutes recollecting the events of the day, starting from the present moment and working backward to when you got up. Then dwell on the happiest periods in your life, from the past and present. Finally practise *Relaxation* (p. 37) until you fall asleep naturally.

If you still have trouble falling asleep don't worry – just practise slow abdominal breathing and be aware of your thoughts and bodily sensations without being anxious to fall asleep. You can also try *Meditation* (p. 40) to quieten your mind further. Even if you don't get to sleep, the deep relaxation will have given you enough rest to cope with the coming day.

Insomnia, like fatigue, may be the result of some other ailment. After many days of not sleeping you should consult your doctor.

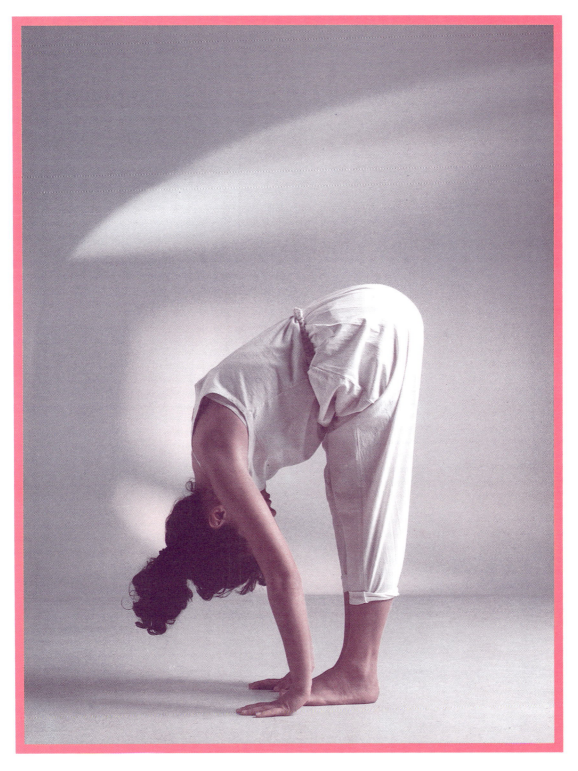

THE HANDS-TO-FEET POSE

OBESITY

The way to lose weight is simple – eat less and exercise more. If you have been obese since childhood or have a strong tendency to over-weight, you may find it more difficult to slim down. Success will follow, though, if you make your energy intake (or food) less than the energy you use to work, live, and exercise. In a few cases obesity may be caused by hor-monal problems needing medical treatment, in which case you should consult your doctor.

A low-calorie, high-fibre diet is the best for losing weight. Maintaining such a diet over long periods, however, can be difficult – especially if you have become habituated to overeating. This is caused by the mind, which craves food as a source of comfort or pleasure. Yoga can help you control your eating habits by giving you mastery over your mind. Relax-ation builds up an inner self-mastery and reduces cravings, while the autosuggestion techniques described below can give relief from the urge to eat.

When you feel a craving for food, say to your-self: "My dear mind, my dear tongue, I am going to eat – but why hurry? Be slow, be easy – let me enjoy this food." Then take five deep breaths and start to eat slowly, savouring the flavours in each morsel.

Alternatively, say: "Eating this food makes me happy, but what it really does is to trigger an inner state of mind – the silence of satis-faction. Therefore I will eat slowly and hold on to that satisfaction instead of gulping my food down quickly."

Yoga is also an ideal form of exercise if you are overweight. It is gentle and carefully graded, reducing the chances of fatigue and injury, and avoids strain to your heart.

FROM THE BASIC SESSION
● Emphasize: *Before You Start; Asanas.*
○ Avoid: *Half Shoulderstand; Shoulderstand; Plough.*
FROM THE AILMENTS SECTION
⊕ Add: *Inverted Corpse (p. 62).*

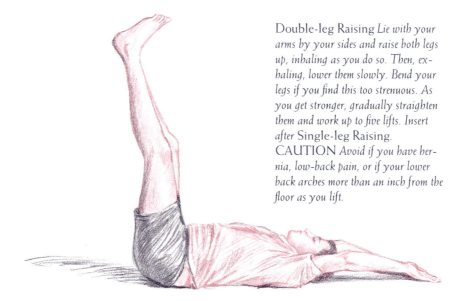

Double-leg Raising *Lie with your arms by your sides and raise both legs up, inhaling as you do so. Then, ex-haling, lower them slowly. Bend your legs if you find this too strenuous. As you get stronger, gradually straighten them and work up to five lifts. Insert after* Single-leg Raising.
CAUTION *Avoid if you have her-nia, low-back pain, or if your lower back arches more than an inch from the floor as you lift.*

CANCER AND AIDS

AIDS is caused by a virus which attacks the immune cells that defend against disease. At the time of writing there is no effective vaccine against or medical treatment for AIDS, but infection stemming from unsafe sexual practices or drug abuse is within your power to prevent, and if you have any doubts you should consult your doctor. Though the virus may remain dormant for many years, once full-blown AIDS develops life expectancy is much reduced. It is at this stage that yoga may provide some help, prolonging life by making the healthy immune cells more effective. It may also help delay the onset of full-blown AIDS in some cases.

Cancer can be caused by many factors and your exposure to them is not always within your control. Nevertheless, you can prevent many cancers by changing your lifestyle and habits. Smoking, alcoholism, and chronic constipation are all cancer-inducing, for example, and stress is also implicated. By practising yoga you can learn to ignore the mind's craving for pleasure through harmful activities and thus avoid such risk factors. In addition, your stress levels will be reduced and your diet will become healthier.

If cancer does develop, yoga can be a useful adjunct to surgery, chemotherapy, and radiotherapy. It can also aid rehabilitation after surgery, but you must first consult a yoga specialist or doctor.

Although not a cure for either cancer or AIDS, yogic attitudes and yogic philosophy can help you face more positively the many emotional and physical trials that both these illnesses bring, while *Yoga Nidra* (below) helps you deal with pain and distress. During *Yoga Nidra*, for both cancer and AIDS, visualize your immune cells being vitalized and attacking the diseased cells. During chemotherapy, the resolve and deep relaxation achieved in *Yoga Nidra* can reduce nausea and other symptoms, and you can visualize your own cells helping the chemicals to do their work and fighting off the cancer.

YOGA NIDRA

Do this whenever you have between 20 and 40 minutes to spare. Make it a healing technique by visualizing positive energy flowing to your body (or negative energy flowing from it) while you are deeply relaxed. Before you start, read *Deep Relaxation Technique (DRT)* on page 37. Familiarize yourself with this, and then start as in *DRT* and follow the instructions below. Try not to fall asleep as you relax.

Make a carefully chosen resolve, such as "I will get better and make a positive contribution to those around me." Then, do the sequence given on page 37. Next, observe your breath passing through your nostrils or your chest, or in an imaginary passage between your navel and your throat. Just be aware; don't try to control it. This promotes relaxation and concentration, and awakens vitalizing energies. Then, move your awareness to your emotions and sensations. Think of pairs of opposites, such as hot/cold, heavy/light, pain/pleasure, joy/sorrow, love/hate. This brings relaxation and control on the plane of feelings and emotions. Now, visualize a series of images or symbols, for example a landscape, oceans, mountains, flowers, holy people, or a religious symbol. End by repeating the resolve you made at the start and slowly return to a more active state.

There are many variations of *Yoga Nidra*, some of which are available in other books and audio cassettes (see Resources p. 95).

CIRCULATION

Your heart is the hardest-working muscle in your body. It is constantly busy, pumping blood through your arteries and veins and thus providing all your tissues with adequate nourishment, oxygen supply, and a means of disposing of wastes. This system is remarkably resilient but continued abuse through smoking, stress, obesity, high cholesterol intake, uncontrolled diabetes, and lack of exercise can lead to degenerative diseases, such as heart disease. These are the most common cause of premature debilitation and death in affluent societies but they can usually be avoided by reducing the principal risk factors.

Yoga is extremely useful in the treatment and management of these conditions. Yogis can manipulate their heart rate at will, and even people with no prior experience of yoga can soon learn to reduce high blood pressure. By working on both your mind and body, yoga teaches you to change your attitudes and reduce stress, while at the same time strengthening your organs. Yogic relaxation and psychology also help you to develop the self-discipline you need to reduce the risk factors in your lifestyle.

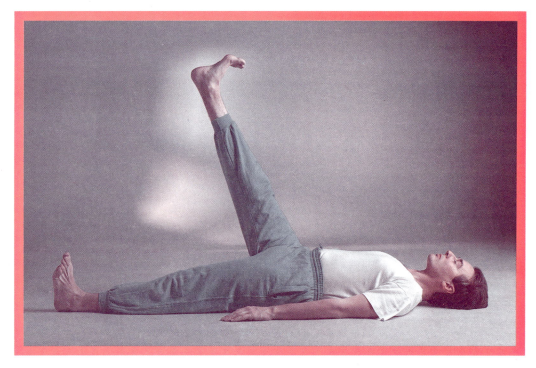

SINGLE-LEG RAISING

HYPERTENSION

Blood pressure varies according to your degree of arousal. When you are calm, it is low, but it rises when you feel excited or when you are under stress. This is brought about by the action of the sympathetic nervous system, which makes the muscles in the artery walls contract in response to stimulation.

Constant high blood pressure (HBP), or hypertension, occurs after long periods of overstimulation, when your arteries become habituated to constant contraction. Though there may be no symptoms initially, it is important to control HBP, since it may eventually damage the brain and other vital organs if left untreated.

Sometimes hypertension results from causes other than stress, so consult your doctor before starting yoga therapy. Yoga can have a supporting effect, if drug therapy is prescribed or surgery is performed. If the cause is stress, practise yoga daily: concentrate on reducing stress reactions, avoid excessive stimulation, and cultivate yogic attitudes in everyday life. But avoid all inverted postures.

FROM THE BASIC SESSION
● Emphasize: *Breathe and Stretch; Relaxation; Pranayama; Meditation; Emotion Culturing.*
○ Avoid: *Loosening Up; Sun Salute; Prone Asanas; Supine Asanas; Moon; Rapid Abdominal Breathing.*

HEART DISEASE

Clogging of the arteries is part of a natural ageing process that begins in childhood, but the speed of modern life and your lifestyle can accelerate the changes. Degeneration of the arteries restricts the flow of blood to the heart muscles, which become starved of oxygen. This causes angina and can lead to heart attacks, where a blood clot forms and completely blocks the flow of blood to the heart. As a consequence, parts of the heart's muscles die through lack of oxygen.

If you can stop smoking, reduce stress and cholesterol, and bring factors such as hypertension, high blood sugar, and obesity under control, you greatly reduce your chances of developing heart disease. These risk factors all have a common base – the mind obtaining pleasure at the expense of health and well-

being. Your need for reward, either through success at work or through excessive indulgence, ceases to be under your control and starts to control you instead. This reflects an inner unrest that yoga can help you rectify.

Relaxation will immediately reduce stress levels, while at a more fundamental level *Happiness Analysis* (p. 13) will change your attitudes, free you from dependency on health-damaging activities, and help you find contentment from within.

FROM THE BASIC SESSION
● Emphasize: *Relaxation; Pranayama; Meditation; Emotion Culturing.*
○ Avoid: *Loosening Up; Locust; Bow; Supine Asanas.*
FROM THE AILMENTS SECTION
⊕ Add: *Cyclic Meditation (pp. 54-5)*

VARICOSE VEINS

Like many other conditions, varicose veins are more easily prevented than cured. They are caused by the heart's inability to maintain the flow of blood. Circulation in the veins is usually aided by muscular activity, such as walking, but if you are inactive blood may accumulate in the legs, causing the veins to stretch and elongate. This results in chronic pain, discoloration of the skin, and repeated nonhealing ulcers. More serious complications can occur if a clot forms in the stagnant blood and moves up into the heart or lungs. Yoga can help you avoid clots by making you fit and active, stimulating circulation, and improving blood drainage.

Once varicose veins are formed, yoga cannot cure them; the shape, size, and appearance of the veins under the skin will remain the same. It does, however, help you mitigate the symptoms and prevent further deterioration. Most useful are the inverted postures,

such as the *Shoulderstand* (p. 31), which improve drainage and reduce stagnation of the blood in your limbs.

Before you start yoga, however, consult your doctor and make sure that no clots have formed in your deep veins. Though yoga might reduce your tendency to form clots, if one is already there it may be dislodged by certain yoga exercises or movements. Until you get clearance from your doctor, avoid *Loosening Up* (pp. 22-3), *Sun Salute* (pp. 24-5), and all the *Asanas* (pp. 26-35).
CAUTION Do not follow the guidelines given below without consulting your doctor.

FROM THE BASIC SESSION
● Emphasize: *Breathe and Stretch; Half Shoulderstand; Shoulderstand; Plough; Fish; Pranayama.*
○ Avoid: *Jogging.*
FROM THE AILMENTS SECTION
⊕ Add: *Inverted Corpse (below).*

Inverted Corpse *Lie near a wall and raise your legs, resting them on the wall either vertically or at a 45° angle, without bending your knees. You may, if you prefer, place a cushion under your buttocks, but not during menstruation. Relax. Practise after the Prone Asanas or during the day.*
CAUTION *Avoid if you have recently formed clots in your veins or if you have hypertension.*

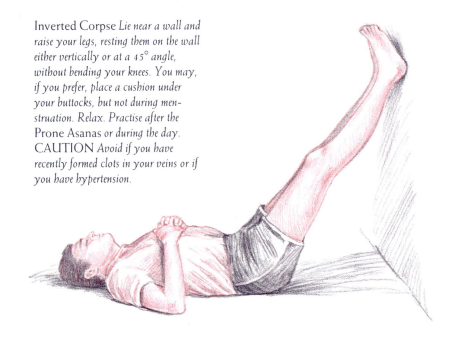

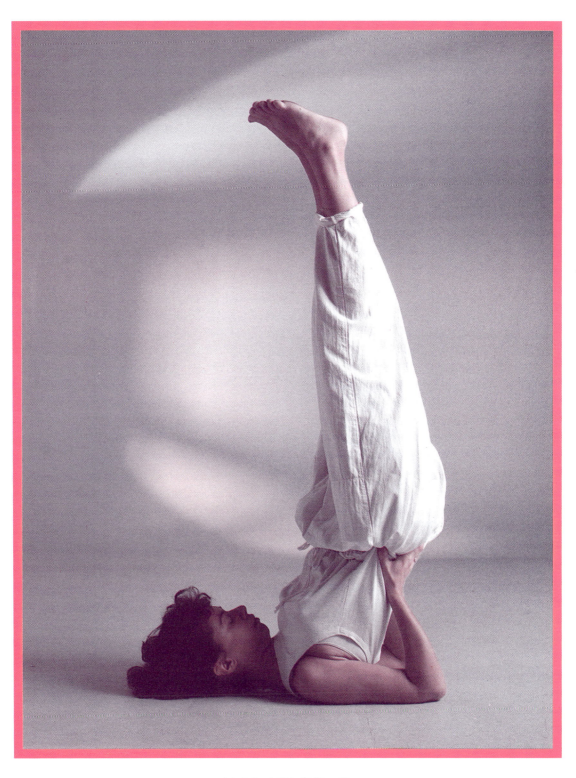

THE SHOULDERSTAND

Respiration

Breathing sustains life, but natural breathing brings health, happiness, and renewal as well. It clears the mind and calms the emotions, and releases the vitalizing flow of energy within you. Yet many of us have lost the capacity to breathe healthily. Sedentary living and mental and emotional stress have all taken their toll, leading to shallow, irregular breathing that can affect our moods from day to day and our health in the long term. Chronic fatigue, respiratory infections, and many allergies can be caused by bad breathing habits. Perhaps the greatest contribution that yoga will make to your well-being is to retrain you to breathe naturally.

Many people with serious respiratory ailments have found a solution in yoga. As the mind is calmed the hyper-reactivity that causes diseases such as bronchial asthma and nasal allergy is reduced. Yoga also strengthens your immune system, so chronic infections are less likely. Finally, if your lungs are permanently damaged, as in chronic bronchitis, yoga teaches you how to improve the mechanical efficiency of your breathing and make the most of your lung capacity (and also helps you to give up smoking).

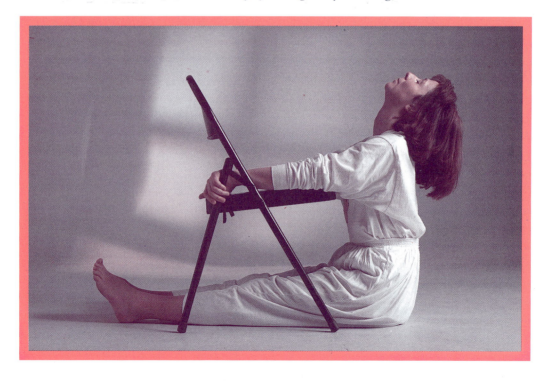

CHAIR BREATHING

NASAL ALLERGY

As well as being the organ of smell, your nose acts as your body's personal built-in aircon-ditioner; it filters, warms, and humidifies the air as you breathe in, before it goes down into your lungs.

The sneezing reflex is also part of this pro-tective system, used to expel foreign irritant substances that enter as you inhale. As soon as these touch the nasal lining, nervous signals are sent off to the brain, which then initiates the sneezing reflex, sending a violent blast of air through the nose. This is followed by a swelling of the nasal lining that blocks the passage and also the copious secretion of fluid, which washes out the irritant and prevents it re-entering the respiratory tract.

Nasal allergy, characterized by excessive sneezing and a continuously runny or blocked nose, occurs when this response becomes over-reactive. It can be triggered by many agents, such as pollen or house dust, or by intrinsic mental factors, such as emotional conflict or oversensitivity.

Yoga can help you increase the nasal lining's tolerance to these agents through simple breathing exercises, *asanas*, and the yogic *Nasal Wash* below. Do the *Nasal Wash* before your daily session, and up to three times a day when your nose is blocked or runny. Patients have consistently observed a marked improve-ment, even within two to four weeks, though the level of allergens in their surroundings remained the same. This indicates that, all too often, nasal allergy is simply a sign of hyper-reactivity, without fundamental physical causes underlying it.

FROM THE BASIC SESSION
● Emphasize: *Breathe and Stretch; Jogging; Rapid Abdominal Breathing.*
FROM THE AILMENTS SECTION
⊕ Add: *Forced Alternate-nostril Breathing (p. 70).*

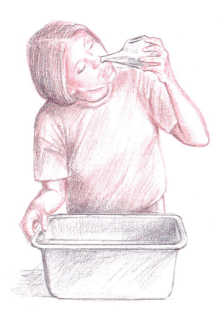

Nasal Wash *Fill a pot with a spout with lightly salted, lukewarm water (use one teaspoon salt/pint). Tilt your head to the left, and insert the spout into your right nostril. Pour water into this slowly, so it comes out of your left nos-tril. Repeat on the other side. Blow out any remaining water, one nostril at a time. Next, tilt your head backward and pour water up your right nostril so it runs into your mouth, then spit it out. Repeat for the left. Use one teacup of water for every nostril wash. Practise up to three times a day, once before your yoga session.*

BRONCHIAL ASTHMA

Your lungs are intricately designed and regulated to suit your ever-changing needs. Your windpipe divides and redivides into smaller and smaller tubes known as bronchi and bronchioles. These eventually lead to tiny air sacs, or alveoli, where oxygen in the air you breathe in is exchanged for carbon dioxide in your blood. In order to reach the air sacs, however, the air must first pass through the entire bronchial "tree". The amount of air you get is regulated before it reaches the air sacs, by altering the width of the bronchial tubes.

The walls of the bronchial tubes contain rings of muscle that can expand or contract them. These muscles are controlled by the brain via the involuntary nervous system. This consists of the sympathetic nerves, which dilate the bronchial tubes, and the parasympathetic nerves, which constrict them. When you are active, and therefore need a lot of oxygen, the brain sends messages that cause the bronchial tubes to dilate, allowing more air to enter. When you are inactive and need less oxygen, your brain constricts the bronchial tubes, so less air can enter.

During an asthmatic attack, this response no longer works properly. The bronchial walls are constricted inappropriately, leading to a shortage of oxygen supply to the blood. But the constriction is temporary and the lungs return to normal after the attack, so there is no physical damage to their structure. Asthma is, therefore, reversible and in principle it can be completely controlled.

This excessive narrowing of the bronchi, or "bronchoconstriction", happens when the parasympathetic nerves are overstimulated. Air flow is further restricted by irritation of the bronchial walls, which leads to swelling of the lining of the bronchi and to the secretion of mucus. Also, it is a common – and natural – response for asthmatics to actively tighten their chest muscles during an attack, in an attempt to inhale more air, and to be afraid of exhaling. This panicking acts to make breathing even more difficult than it already is.

Attacks can be triggered by many factors, both physical and psychological. They can be brought about by exercise, excitement, cold air, and infections and also can be triggered by specific substances, for example pollen, and the tiny mites that live in animal fur and house dust. If you become allergic to one of these, your body regards the allergen as dangerous. Certain cells on the bronchial lining react to its presence by releasing chemicals that irritate the mucus-producing cells and the parasympathetic nerves. And the brain responds to the impulses from the parasympathetic nerves by stimulating them more, making the bronchoconstriction even worse.

Asthmatic attacks can also be triggered by the brain on its own. Just seeing an image of a hayfield can set off an attack in a person allergic to hay; and strong, suppressed emotions can also induce an attack. Asthmatics are often highly sensitive and deeply emotional people, who frequently find it difficult to express their feelings.

Though conventional treatment for asthma does exist, it consists mainly of symptom-controlling medication. Bronchodilators expand the bronchi and immunosuppressors block the allergic reaction; but neither of these treatments can cure asthma, they can only control it. And often their effectiveness diminishes with time, so increasingly larger dosages, or more powerful drugs, are needed, and side-effects become more severe.

ASTHMA AND YOGA THERAPY

Yoga therapy aims to cure asthma, not just control it. The treatment works on different levels: physical, mental, emotional, and through releasing the flow of energy. Each aspect of yoga practice in the *Basic Session* brings its own benefits; the stamina of your respiratory system increases, mucus is drained from your lungs, you learn to use your lungs properly, and the tense muscles in your chest are relaxed. As well, energy blocks are released, your energy levels rise, and your body and mind are calmed and harmonized. *Emotion Culturing* (p. 41) and *Happiness Analysis* (p. 13) then help to reduce negative upsurges.

Yoga also reduces the allergic response in your lungs, though how this comes about is not yet known. Another useful benefit of yoga is the increasing mastery that you gain over your involuntary nervous reflexes. This enables you to reduce the overactivity of the parasympathetic nerves, and to react less to factors that normally trigger an attack.

As well as making attacks less frequent, yoga can assist you during an attack. The increased capacity to relax and to control your breathing enables you to avoid panic and thus reduce the attack's severity. To avoid an impending attack, practise *Chair Breathing*, outlined on pages 68–9. Start when you feel an attack beginning, letting the sequence relax you.

Practise the whole of the *Basic Session*, as modified below, but take care not to strain yourself with the more active exercises. If you practise for one hour each day, you should see some benefits within a few days. For the maximum effect, however, you may have to continue for a year or two, especially if your asthma is severe.

FROM THE BASIC SESSION

● Emphasize: *Before You Start; Triangle; Cobra; Bow; Shoulderstand; Fish; Forward Stretch; Supine Kneebend; Pranayama; Emotion Culturing.*

FROM THE AILMENTS SECTION

⊕ Add: *Butterfly* (p. 79).

BENEFITS OF YOGA

The gentle breathing exercises in *Breathe and Stretch* (pp. 20–1) and *Jogging* (p. 22) help to make your respiratory system more robust and make you more energetic. The *Asanas* (pp. 26–35), relax the tense muscles in your chest, so you can breathe more easily, and release energy blocks. Inverted *asanas* also drain mucus from your lungs. *Meditation* (p. 40) helps to calm you and harmonizes your mind and your body. *Pranayama* also brings many benefits (see opposite).

CHILDREN AND ASTHMA

Yoga can help young children suffering from asthma. But for yoga therapy to be successful, it is vital that they practise the *Basic Session* every day. It is hard for young children to develop the application that is needed without proper encouragement. Practise with children daily, making the session fun, and giving them a sense of security. When your child has an attack, guide him/her through *Chair Breathing* (pp. 68–9).

PRANAYAMA AND ASTHMA

Pranayama (pp. 38–9) brings deeper benefits than the simple mechanical effect of exercising the lungs. *Sectional Breathing* teaches you to use every part of your lungs, and *Rapid Abdominal Breathing* stimulates your lung tissues, relaxes your chest muscles, and energizes your whole system. *Alternate-nostril Breathing* has a calming effect, working with meditation to bring you harmony and peace.

CHAIR BREATHING

You can practise this sequence during an asthma attack, ideally when it is just starting. It helps to reduce the attack's severity and may reduce (or eliminate) your need for drugs to release bronchospasm (p. 65). Initially, it takes about 30 to 45 minutes but with practice, it will only need about 20 minutes. As you practise *Chair Breathing*, try to relax and calm your mind.
CAUTION Omit *Moon Breathing* and *Forward-backward Bending* during menstruation, or if you have hypertension or glaucoma.

1 Head Down *Sit on a mat in front of a chair with your legs outstretched. Pull the chair toward your chest, and collapse your head and arms on to its seat. Tighten your entire body from toes to head, then relax each part locally. Now, move your head backward and forward slowly five times. Then, repeat another five times, but this time inhale as deeply and slowly as you can as your head goes back and exhale as it comes forward. Next, move your head back and forth five times as before, but chant "AH" in a low tone while coming forward, synchronizing the sound with the movement. Then, finish by repeating the previous sequence five times again, but chanting "MM" instead of "AH".*

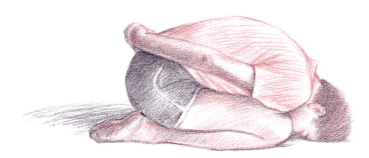

2 Moon Breathing *Kneel and sit on your heels. Keep your spine erect. Now, move your head forward and back five times and then five times again, but this time inhale as it goes back and exhale as it comes forward. Next, grasp your right wrist with your left hand, behind your back. As you inhale, move your head back and relax your neck muscles. Then, exhaling, bend forward until your head rests on the ground in front of your knees. If this is difficult, rest your head on top of your knees or on a cushion. Repeat five times, synchronizing each breath with the movement. Then, repeat another five times, but chant "MM" as you go down.*

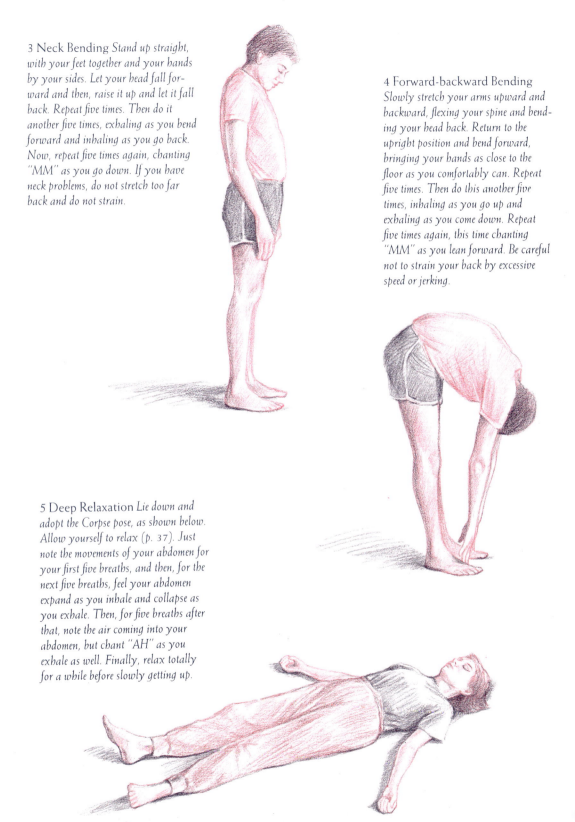

3 Neck Bending *Stand up straight, with your feet together and your hands by your sides. Let your head fall forward and then, raise it up and let it fall back. Repeat five times. Then do it another five times, exhaling as you bend forward and inhaling as you go back. Now, repeat five times again, chanting "MM" as you go down. If you have neck problems, do not stretch too far back and do not strain.*

4 Forward-backward Bending *Slowly stretch your arms upward and backward, flexing your spine and bending your head back. Return to the upright position and bend forward, bringing your hands as close to the floor as you comfortably can. Repeat five times. Then do this another five times, inhaling as you go up and exhaling as you come down. Repeat five times again, this time chanting "MM" as you lean forward. Be careful not to strain your back by excessive speed or jerking.*

5 Deep Relaxation *Lie down and adopt the Corpse pose, as shown below. Allow yourself to relax (p. 37). Just note the movements of your abdomen for your first five breaths, and then, for the next five breaths, feel your abdomen expand as you inhale and collapse as you exhale. Then, for five breaths after that, note the air coming into your abdomen, but chant "AH" as you exhale as well. Finally, relax totally for a while before slowly getting up.*

COLDS AND SINUSITIS

Colds are viral infections that may afflict anyone. Most of us get a cold at least once a year, yet despite much research there is still no effective vaccine or cure. You can obtain some relief by treating cold symptoms with drugs but these do not usually hasten recovery or aid your natural healing processes. Though colds are rarely serious, they often lower your resistance to bacterial infections.

In sinusitis, for example, the excess mucus produced by a cold is infected by bacteria that then spread to the sinuses. When this happens your mucous membranes become inflamed and your sinuses fill with mucus and pus. This leads to headaches, loss of the sense of smell, and possibly pain. Colds often trigger sinusitis because the sinuses are connected to the nasal passages, but it can also be caused by allergic reactions and is exacerbated by emotional tensions and stress.

Yoga can help you to reduce the frequency and intensity of both these ailments. The *Basic Session*, as modified below, gives a boost to your immune system, so you are less likely to succumb to infection. *Sectional Breathing* and *Rapid Abdominal Breathing* (pp. 38–9) increase the resistance of your respiratory tract, and *Nasal Wash* (p. 65) and *Forced Alternate-nostril Breathing* (below) increase the resistance of your sinuses. But if you have a fever, avoid all exercises in *Before You Start*, all *Asanas*, and *Rapid Abdominal Breathing*. Practise gentle *Pranayama* (pp. 38–9), *DRT* (p. 37), and *Yoga Nidra* (p. 59) while lying or sitting in bed.

FROM THE BASIC SESSION
● Emphasize: *Breathe and Stretch; Jogging; Pranayama.*
FROM THE AILMENTS SECTION
⊕ Add: *Forced Alternate-nostril Breathing (below).*

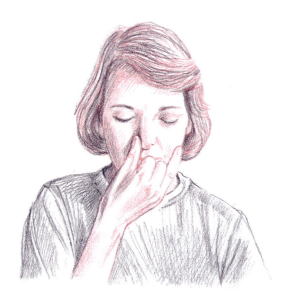

Forced Alternate-nostril Breath-ing *For this exercise you must combine the techniques for* Alternate-nostril Breathing *and* Rapid Abdominal Breathing *(see p. 39). Breathe out through alternate nostrils, using the same hand positions, as in* Alternate-nostril Breathing. *But breathe in through both nostrils at once, and exhale sharply by using your abdomi-nal muscles – as for* Rapid Abdomi-nal Breathing. *Do several rounds but be careful not to strain your ears by exhaling too forcefully. Do with the other* Pranayama *exercises.*
CAUTION *Avoid during menstrua-tion and if you have hypertension or epilepsy.*

CHRONIC LUNG DISEASES

Your body contains many structures that, had they been manufactured, would be regarded as the pinnacles of human achievement. None more so, perhaps, than your lungs, whose extraordinary design allows them to pack an area the size of a tennis court in the small space between your ribs.

Starting with the division of the right and left bronchi to each lung, the air passages divide and redivide into ever smaller tubes that end in clusters of alveoli, or air sacs. These minute globular air sacs have just the right shape to promote circulation of gases and the exchange of oxygen and carbon dioxide in the bloodstream, while systems of muscles regulate the width of the air passages, so just the right amount of air enters the lungs. These are just a few of the characteristics that combine to allow your lungs to work efficiently and appropriately, depending on your activities.

Yet we often become too familiar with these natural miracles of design, forgetting that they cannot be matched or replaced once damaged. We abuse our bodies, and the incredible structures that keep us alive and healthy, until neither our natural healing processes nor medical expertise can heal us. And while some causes of permanent damage, such as infections and accidents, are not within our immediate control, others are, including smoking and the general degradation of the immune system that results from an unhealthy diet and lifestyle.

Chronic bronchitis and emphysema are two lung disorders that are often a result of smoking. Cigarette smoke and tar irritate and damage the inner lining of the bronchi, leading to early morning cough, large amounts of phlegm in the lungs, and possibly wheezing. After a few years the air sacs in the lung become permanently distended, decreasing their active surface area and also impeding the flow of air through the lungs. This condition, called emphysema, causes severe breathlessness on exertion.

Other chronic lung diseases are immune-related disorders, such as sarcoidosis, allergic inflammation of the air sacs, and occupational lung diseases caused by exposure to harmful or poisonous substances. Some lung infections, such as tuberculosis and fungus infection cause damage such as lung abscesses and dilation of the bronchial tubes unless they are quickly cured or controlled.

Yoga cannot repair lung damage once it has occurred, but it can help you manage such ailments and enhances the effectiveness of surgical, drug, and physiotherapy treatments. Yogic breathing techniques and *asanas* teach you how to oxygenate all parts of your lungs, open out blocked air passages, and expand partially collapsed lungs. They also promote the drainage of secretions and improve general health and stamina. As the efficiency of your immune system increases, infections clear up more quickly and drugs become more effective, so smaller doses are required.

In addition to physical improvement through yogic *asanas* and breathing, which increase functional lung capacity and act to minimize the degree of damage, yoga makes another important contribution. As a technique for mastery over the mind, yoga can help you to give up smoking. This is vital in the case of severe lung damage, such as in chronic bronchitis and emphysema.

FROM THE BASIC SESSION
● Emphasize: *Pranayama*.
○ Avoid: *Loosening Up*.

DIGESTION

Your digestive system provides your body with energy and the raw materials it needs to grow and maintain itself. Your sense of taste and smell help you select nutritious, safe foods and the food you eat is converted into an absorbable form by chewing and chemical action. Nutrients then pass into your bloodstream, and from there to your cells, while roughage and waste are excreted through your anus. Most of this process is governed by the autonomic nervous system and is outside your conscious control.

The body normally rests after eating, allowing extra blood to go to the digestive system. In emergencies, blood is diverted from digestion to the muscles and organs of action. If you are subjected to chronic stress and have an unbalanced lifestyle, your body can forget how to relax and your natural rhythms and energy flows become disturbed. This leads to many types of digestive disorders. Yoga can help improve, and even correct, many digestive ailments by reducing stress and balancing your energies. It also encourages you to adopt a sound diet and healthy eating habits, which are the basis of a healthy digestive system.

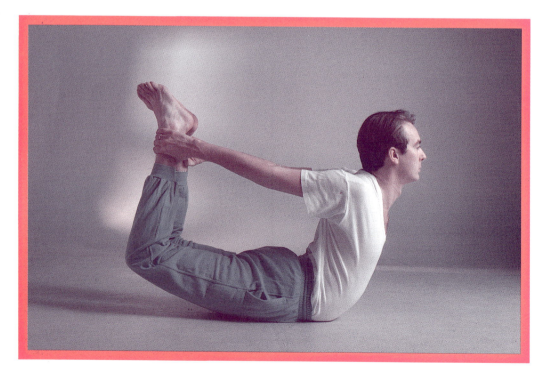

THE BOW

DIARRHOEA

When you are healthy, your body naturally follows a regular cycle of bowel action and your stools are long and firm, though not hard. Diarrhoea, where faeces become almost liquid and bowel action is speeded up, can be caused by many factors, ranging from serious ailments to eating laxative foods. Regular bouts of diarrhoea, or even persistent diarrhoea, are often related to stress, however, and can be cured by yoga.

IRRITABLE BOWEL SYNDROME (IBS)

The movement of food through your bowels is controlled by the autonomic nervous system, supervised by the hypothalamus in the brain. This means that bowel action can be affected by your mental state and many bowel disorders occur as a result of stress. When such conditions become severe and chronic they are known as IBS or irritable bowel syndrome. IBS can manifest itself as persistent diarrhoea, chronic constipation, or alternating bouts of each condition.

Several different factors are thought to contribute to IBS, such as lack of time to sit on the toilet and relax the bowels, lack of exercise, irregular eating habits, refined foods, food additives, and phobias. And there is no effective medical treatment; doctors usually recommend a combination of diet and exercise but this often fails since it does not address the underlying cause of IBS.

In yogic terms, IBS can be explained as a disturbance in the flow of *prana*, or life-energy (pp. 10–11). This has three forms; an upward flow (*Udana*), a downward flow (*Apana*), and a balancing movement around the navel (*Samana*). Diarrhoea is caused by an excessive release of *Apana* and alternating diarrhoea and constipation by a disturbance in *Samana*.

Yoga usually brings improvement within a few weeks, and can sometimes cure IBS completely in several months. Modify the *Basic Session* using the advice box below, and for best results practise at least 30 minutes a day. In general, inverted postures help stem the release of *Apana* and therefore improve diarrhoea, while deep relaxation in *Pranayama* (pp. 38–9) will help to stabilize the *Samana*. DRT (p. 37), *Pranayama*, and *Meditation* (p. 40) also help to harmonize the energy flows and to reduce anxiety and nervousness, which is often associated with diarrhoea.

A change in diet is also called for; eat bland food at first, but as the diarrhoea abates shift to whole foods containing lots of natural fibre, fresh fruit, and vegetables. Try to establish regular and relaxed mealtimes (pp. 42–3).

ULCERATIVE COLITIS

This is a serious colonic disease that leads to ulcers in the bowel wall and its symptoms include bloody diarrhoea with mucus, and pain. It occurs because of an alteration in the immune resistance of the inner bowel lining and if untreated can lead to fatal bleeding, colonic paralysis, rupture, or cancer. Consult your doctor immediately if you suspect that you may have this disorder.

Like IBS, ulcerative colitis is a psychosomatic ailment, often caused by stress, though food allergies may also be involved. The yogic therapy is the same as for IBS (see advice box below), but you should also try to identify what foods you are allergic to, if any, and consult your doctor at regular intervals.

FROM THE BASIC SESSION
● Emphasize: *Half Shoulderstand; Relaxation; Pranayama; Meditation; Emotion Culturing.*

HYPERACIDITY

Every time you eat, your stomach secretes a highly acidic gastric juice, needed for the digestion of food. This secretion is triggered by the vagus nerve – a branch of the parasympathetic nervous system – and is easily exaggerated by stress or strong emotions, such as anger or jealousy. This leads to hyperacidity, a condition where the stomach produces too much gastric juice and damages its own wall.

Your stomach is protected from this acid by a slimy coating of mucin, secreted by its inner lining. The health of the stomach wall is maintained by a very delicate balance of three factors: the blood supply to the wall; the quantity of acid; and the quantity and quality of the mucin coat.

Stress attacks this balance in a number of ways. It makes the vagus nerve hyperactive, so too much acid is produced. It also decreases the blood supply to the stomach wall, which alters the quality of mucin, making the stomach wall more vulnerable to the highly acid fluids. Eventually this process can lead to ulcers in the stomach wall.

Both hyperacidity and ulcers are often found in sedentary workers who take little exercise, eat at irregular times, and work to targets and deadlines.

The yogic approach of holistic therapy, through your body, mind, energy flows, and attitudes, calms your nerves and reduces the number of nervous stimuli to the stomach and improves the blood supply to the stomach wall. As a healthy balance is restored the inflammation is reduced and this allows ulcers to heal naturally.

FROM THE BASIC SESSION
● Emphasize: *Loosening Up; Sun Salute; Standing Asanas; Alternate-nostril Breathing; Emotion Culturing; Yogic Diet.*
○ Avoid: *Sitting Asanas.*
FROM THE AILMENTS SECTION
⊕ Add: *Abdominal Lock (below).*

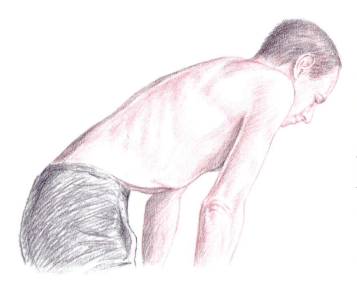

Abdominal Lock *Bend forward and exhale completely through your mouth, then close your throat so no air can enter. Expand your chest, as though inhaling, and suck in your abdomen, forming a deep hollow. Try to relax the muscles as you do so. This may be difficult, but with daily practice you will soon master it. Hold until you need to take a breath, then release and inhale slowly. Insert after* Relaxation.
CAUTION *Avoid during menstruation, pregnancy, active inflammation or bleeding, or if you have hypertension or heart disease.*

HAEMORRHOIDS

Yoga can help you prevent piles, or haemor-rhoids, by promoting local circulation to the anus and reducing constipation. Piles occur when the flow of blood in the anal veins is obstructed, causing them to stretch and elon-gate. If blood drainage is blocked, by chronic constipation for example, piles result.

Sometimes, they can also be a sign of liver disease so consult your doctor before starting yoga. If they are not, treat them by curing constipation and improving drainage from the veins. Read *Constipation* below and combine the practices outlined there with those in the advice box. But avoid *Jogging* (p. 23).

To improve blood drainage practise the *Half Shoulderstand* (p. 31) three times a day, for ten minutes each time. Breathe deeply from your abdomen as you hold the position and con-tract the anus at each exhalation.

Yoga cannot cure already enlarged, non-collapsing piles: these must be dealt with sur-gically. In mild cases, however, it can help you stop the condition deteriorating and relieves unpleasant symptoms. It will also help to prevent any relapse after surgery.

FROM THE BASIC SESSION
- Emphasize: *Half Shoulderstand*.
○ Avoid: *Jogging*
FROM THE AILMENTS SECTION
⊕ Add: *Abdominal Lock* (p. 74); *Abdominal Pumping* (p. 76).

CONSTIPATION

In yoga, bowel disorders are thought to reflect disturbances in the flow of *prana*, or the yogic "life energy". *Prana* has upward flow (*Udana*), downward flow (*Apana*), and a balancing force around the navel (*Samana*) that maintains your normal digestive mobility. Constipation is due to a lack of *Apana*, which can be restored by emphasizing *Standing Asanas* (pp. 27-8). Dis-turbance around the *Samana* causes irregular bowel functions and can be healed by deep relaxation in *Pranayama* (pp. 38-9).

Medically, constipation is another form of IBS, or irritable bowel syndrome (p. 73). In this case your normal bowel movements are slowed down, resulting in the familiar signs of constipation: hard stools, which are difficult to pass, and infrequent bowel clearance. Eat-ing a high-fibre diet, including raw vegetables and fruit, taking regular exercise, and allowing enough time to relax on the toilet are particu-larly useful for dealing with constipation.

Set aside 20 minutes at a fixed time each day and try to develop a daily habit of passing stools. First drink two glasses of luke-warm water and then practise *Rapid Abdominal Breath-ing* (p. 38) while holding the *Half Shoulderstand* (p. 31). Work up to 40 breaths and repeat three times, resting in between. Then, prac-tise the *Embryo* (p 23) and *Jogging* (p. 22). Finally, sit on the toilet and relax.

FROM THE BASIC SESSION
- Emphasize: *Loosening Up; Half Shoulderstand Rapid Abdominal Breathing; Yogic Diet.*

DIABETES

Glucose is your body's energy source and your cells need a steady supply of it to function. It is important, therefore, to regulate your blood glucose level carefully. If it is too low, your cells starve, but a high level, over a long period, leads to infection, muscle wastage, heart attacks, strokes, blindness, or kidney damage. Your glucose levels are kept within safe limits by delicate hormonal control; insulin reduces sugar levels, while glucagon and stress hormones release glucose from your body's energy stores. Diabetes mellitus is diagnosed when, due to hormonal disturbances, blood glucose levels become dangerously high.

There are two forms of diabetes mellitus: insulin-dependent (IDDM) and noninsulin-dependent (NIDDM). The first is due to low insulin-production by the pancreas. The more common type, NIDDM, usually starts after the age of 40 and has many contributory causes, such as obesity, heredity, lack of exercise, autoimmunity, and stress.

Yoga can be a powerful additional tool for enhancing conventional diabetes treatment. It makes diet control and weight reduction easier, and is a good form of exercise. It also reduces stress-hormone levels, improves the function of the pancreas, and normalizes your immune system. In NIDDM, yoga may eliminate your need to take insulin or drugs. In IDDM, however, yoga cannot eliminate your insulin requirement, though it may reduce or stabilize it.

FROM THE BASIC SESSION
● Emphasize: *Bow; Spinal Twist; Relaxation; Pranayama; Meditation; Emotion Culturing.*
FROM THE AILMENTS SECTION
⊕ Add: *Abdominal Lock (p. 74); Abdominal Pumping (below).*

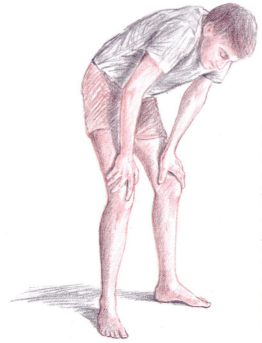

Abdominal Pumping *Lean forward and exhale completely through your mouth. Close your throat so air cannot enter into your lungs. Expand your chest, as if inhaling, and suck your abdomen up into the chest. Then, with your lungs empty, relax your muscles so the abdomen comes out. Suck in the abdomen and pump it in and out until you need to inhale; then breathe normally. Repeat three times. Insert after* Relaxation *and* Abdominal Lock. CAUTION *Avoid during menstruation, pregnancy, active bleeding or inflammation, after surgery, or if you have hypertension or heart disease.*

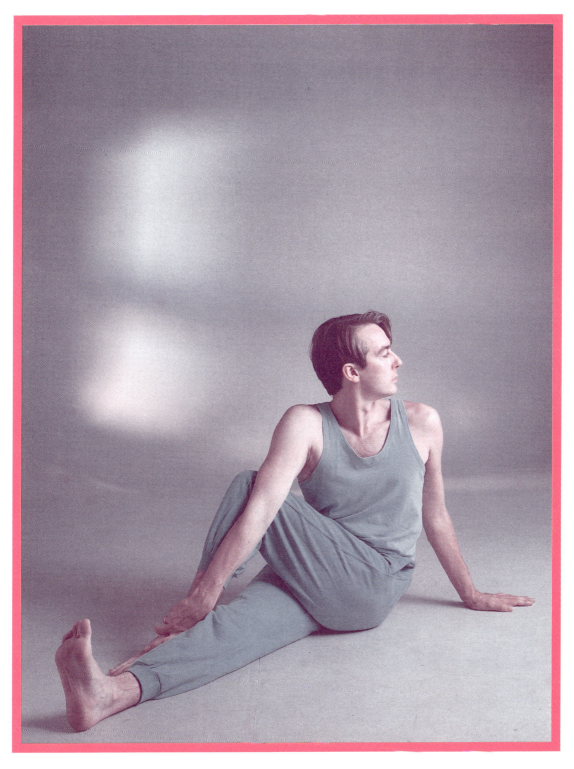

THE SPINAL TWIST

REPRODUCTION

Reproduction brings about the creation of new life. Through participating in this familiar, yet miraculous, process we experience some of the most profound and exhilarating moments in our lives. And just as the reproductive process can affect your entire life, so the way you live, and the attitudes you hold, can affect the reproductive process.

Reproductive problems often have a strong psychosomatic element. Fear, resentment, or guilt over genital functions can cause sexual problems in both sexes; while stress, subconscious needs, and suppressed emotions can bring about many menstrual problems in women. Even physical problems can be exacerbated by the mind. Becoming aware of these hidden factors can help to overcome such ailments.

Yoga helps you to cure yourself holistically, by addressing the mental problems as well as the physical disorder. It slows down the mind and harmonizes negative emotions, promoting your awareness of inner needs and letting you deal with them positively. It can also remove the physical barriers to restoring health, allowing your body to heal itself.

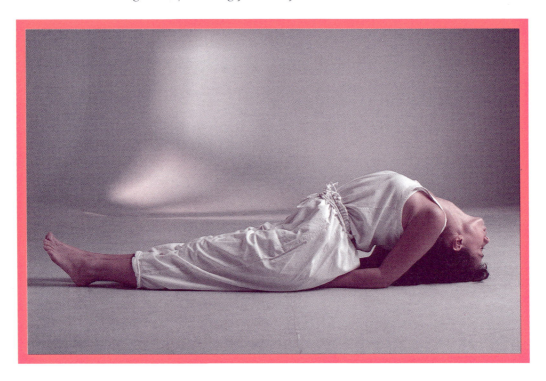

THE FISH

PREMENSTRUAL SYNDROME (PMS)

Many women just before their "period" experience inexplicable mood changes. This phenomenon is called PMS, or premenstrual tension (PMT), and is related to hormone production during the menstrual cycle. It is greatly aggravated by stress, which can influence the production of these hormones. If you have PMS, for up to ten days before menstruation you may feel depressed, anxious, irritable, or afraid – and these feelings can be so intense that they cause disharmony in your relationships, even suicidal tendencies in extreme cases. In yoga, mood fluctuations are seen as manifestations of a distracted mind. Excess energies are being released to flow haphazardly and wastefully, resulting in exhaustion, fatigue, and many other symptoms.

To control these energy surges, practise the *Basic Session* throughout the month. In the last week of your cycle, also practise *DRT* (p. 37) three times a day for 15 minutes each time. If you also experience painful breasts, emphasize the *Camel* (p. 33) but avoid the *Plough* and *Shoulderstand* (p. 31). If you get headaches, try *Neck-rolling* (p. 83) but avoid the *Bow* (p. 30) and the *Moon* (p. 33).

Menopause has similar symptoms to PMS, as well as hot flushes, sweating, insomnia, and muscular pains. If you are 40 years or over, you are approaching menopause and basic yoga, emphasizing *Relaxation* and *Meditation*, will help enormously. Avoid all of *Loosening Up* (pp. 22-3), however, during the first month of yoga. The uterus is particularly sensitive to exercise at this age, and vaginal bleeding may result. Gradually incorporate it as you get used to vigorous movement.

FROM THE BASIC SESSION
● Emphasize: *Triangle; Bow; Half Shoulderstand; Sitting Asanas; Relaxation; Pranayama; Meditation; Emotion Culturing.*
FROM THE AILMENTS SECTION
⊕ Add: *Butterfly (below).*

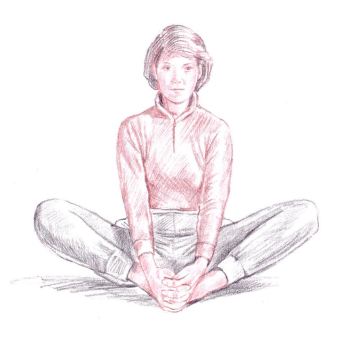

Butterfly *Sit with your spine erect, soles of your feet together, and your heels close to your body. Clasp your feet and gently move your knees up and down. Then, gently lean forward, bending from the hips. Keep your back straight and push from the lower part of your spine. Hold this position for two minutes, feeling the stretch on the inside of the legs. At each breath, relax forward as you exhale, and hold as you inhale. Insert this exercise after the Spinal Twist.*

79

MENSTRUAL PROBLEMS

Menstruation, often known as a "period", is part of the body's preparation for conception and pregnancy. The menstrual cycle is a continuous process that occurs in almost every woman between puberty and menopause and ensures that she is ready to receive and nourish a tiny embryo. At approximately monthly intervals the womb goes through a cycle of growth, cleansing, and regeneration – and it is at the cleansing stage, when the old womb lining is shed, that you have vaginal bleeding.

This cycle is governed by a sensitive hormonal feedback system, initiated by the hypothalamus, a region of the brain. The level of sex hormones fluctuates throughout the month and it is this balance of hormones that governs what happens in your body. When you are healthy and fit and at peace with yourself the cyclic fluctuation of hormones is regular, since the level of one determines the level of another. But emotional turmoil and stress can interfere with this feedback system and result in menstrual problems.

Painful periods of varying intensity occur in most women at some time and slight pain or discomfort are common. In some women, especially if they are young, the symptoms can be more severe, including excessive pain and vomiting. A number of factors can cause pain, such as hormonal irregularities, the position of the uterus, or a narrow cervix. Stress and unexpressed emotions can exacerbate this condition, but in some cases pain can be due to another ailment, so consult a doctor first. Yoga can help to reduce the stress and to normalize hormone levels, thus helping to minimize or eliminate pain.

Heavy and frequent periods at irregular intervals, when they are caused by hormone imbalances, are known as dysfunctional uterine bleeding. The conventional treatment for this condition is hormone therapy – which can have unpleasant side-effects – and if this fails a hysterectomy is often performed. Yoga has helped many women avoid both these alternatives by restoring their hormonal balance naturally, without drugs.

Absence of menstruation, though it can sometimes be due to physical damage, is often caused by emotional and environmental factors. Extreme degrees of anxiety, stress, and strain or abrupt changes in environment can affect the hypothalamus, which is directly linked to the emotion centre in the brain cortex, and block the menstrual cycle. Over-training (for example in athletes) or your weight can also play a part in this disorder.

Yoga helps to release suppressed emotions and relieves anxiety and stress, restoring your emotional stability. *Asanas* such as the *Butterfly* (p. 79) improve the circulation to the pelvic region and send messages to the brain to re-start the cycle. Through yoga your general health improves, your weight normalizes, and yogic deep relaxation gives you a sense of wellbeing – and thus the barriers to restoring the natural cycle are removed.

Practise the *Basic Session*, as modified below, except when you have a period. During your period practise: *Relaxation* (p. 37); *Alternate-nostril Breathing* (p. 39); *Folded-tongue Breathing* (p. 39); *Sounds Breathing* (p. 39); *Meditation* (p. 40); and *Emotion Culturing* (p. 41).

FROM THE BASIC SESSION
● Emphasize: *Hands-to-feet Pose; Triangle; Moon; Forward Stretch; DRT; Pranayama; Meditation; Emotion Culturing.*
FROM THE AILMENTS SECTION
⊕ Add: *Butterfly (p. 79)*

MALE REPRODUCTIVE DISORDERS

The male reproductive organs have two main functions: lovemaking and fertilization and as a urinary tract. Both these functions can be disturbed by psychosomatic factors and stress, as well as the gradual degeneration that accompanies old age.

Stress is a major cause of sexual problems; it makes you less affectionate, less imaginative, and disturbs the harmony between you and your partner, hence disturbing your sexual relationship. It can also often cause premature ejaculation or impotence.

Yoga reduces stress, tones your body, and balances your energy flow, helping you to overcome such problems. *Meditation* and *Emotion Culturing* also help you to understand and relate to your partner better.

To avoid premature ejaculation, practise *Breathe and Stretch* (pp. 20–1) before you go to bed and try to breathe from your abdomen during intercourse to relax yourself. To help impotence and boost flagging sexual energies, emphasize *Before You Start* (pp. 20–5), as well as the practices listed below. For anxiety, read page 86, and to reduce stress, practise *Cyclic Meditation* (pp. 54–5).

In later life, men often suffer from an enlarged prostate gland, which may block the outlet from the bladder. The yoga session recommended below can help to prevent minor blockages. More difficult blockages can sometimes be specifically relieved by doing the *Half Shoulderstand* (p. 31) or the *Supine Butterfly* (below), or by an extremely hot bath. Persistent blockages, reduced flow, and residual urine, however, require surgical treatment.

FROM THE BASIC SESSION
● Emphasize: *Triangle; Shoulderstand; Relaxation; Pranayama; Meditation; Emotion Culturing.*
FROM THE AILMENTS SECTION
⊕ *Add: Butterfly (p. 79); Supine Butterfly (below).*

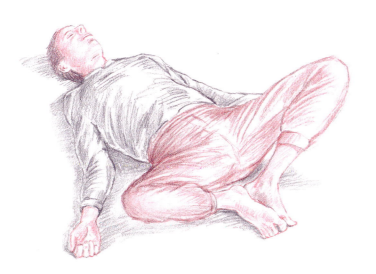

Supine Butterfly *Lie on your back, on a firm, flat surface, with your arms by your sides. Raising your knees, bring your feet as close to your buttocks as you can. Put the soles of your feet against each other, or, if this is difficult, bring the inner side of your soles together but not the outer edge. Relax, letting your knees sink symmetrically down toward the floor. Remain in this position for at least five minutes. You can read or talk while holding this posture to pass the time. This exercise relaxes, and brings blood to the prostate and surrounding tissues. Practise after the* Spinal Twist *and the* Butterfly.

81

NERVOUS SYSTEM

The nervous system is the most complex and highly organized system in the body, and its influence on health and happiness is immense. All basic bodily functions are regulated by it, so any dysfunction can be expressed as a physical or psychiatric disorder. Even the intellect, feelings, and consciousness may be involved in creating the disorganization that leads to disease.

For example, the high incidence of stress-related ailments at this time is partly due to an imbalance between right- and left-brain thinking. The left brain is responsible for logical analysis and language, and its recent development has resulted in the modern scientific revolution. The right brain, however, which is concerned with feelings, intuition, and artistic qualities, has been undervalued. This lopsided development has caused disharmony and stress, which are often expressed as physical disease.

Yoga, being a systematic science of the mind, can provide help for many nervous disorders, from tension headaches to psychiatric disturbances. In fact, yoga works primarily through your mind and nervous system, restoring harmony to their function and thus curing many psychosomatic ailments.

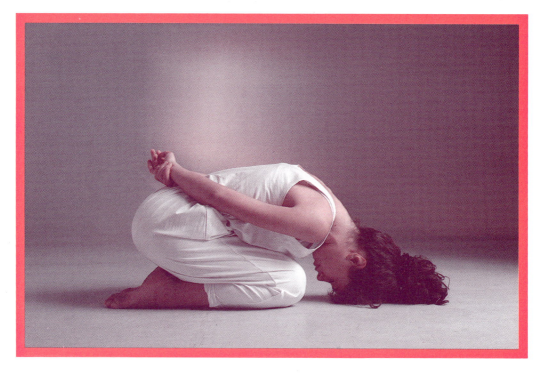

THE MOON

HEADACHES

There are more than a hundred causes of head-ache, some functional and some organic. In some cases, they may indicate a major dis-order, such as brain tumour. If yours are acute or have changed recently you should consult a doctor. Mostly, however, yoga provides an effective alternative to pain killers.

Through *asanas* that calm you, *pranayama* exercises that inhibit random energy flares, and *meditation* that cultivates and relaxes your mind, yoga offers a holistic form of pain relief. It stops you becoming locked in the vicious circle of pain-anxiety-pain that leads to chronic headache problems. Your reaction to a headache changes, which makes it go away more quickly, and as you become calmer, the frequency of your headaches decreases.

Tension headaches are the most common and are caused by constant overcontraction of the neck and head muscles. This is usually the result of emotional or mental conflicts, but in highly sensitive people almost any change in their surroundings may trigger this type of headache. Migraines are more deep-rooted, involving the flow of blood to the brain. Migraine symptoms include pain on one side of the head, nausea, and visual disturbances. It can be triggered by food allergens, sudden stimuli, fatigue, or anxiety.

Yoga is a useful therapy for both of these, as well as headaches caused by eyestrain, sinus-itis, or hangover. But avoid excessive forward or backward bending, which change the press-ure in your head. For direct relief try a *Nasal Wash* (p. 65), deep relaxation (*DRT* – p. 37) with cold pads over your eyes, or *Neck-rolling* (below) three times a day.

FROM THE BASIC SESSION
● Emphasize: *Breathe and Stretch; Relaxation; Pranayama.*
○ Avoid: *Fish; Moon.*
FROM THE AILMENTS SECTION
⊕ Add: *Neck-rolling (below).*

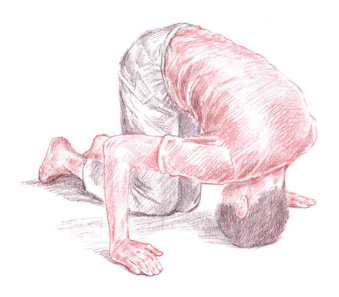

Neck-rolling *Go down on your hands and knees, with your hands under your shoulders. Bend your arms and touch the top of your head on the floor. Then, exhaling, carefully roll your head forward until you feel a gentle stretch along the back of your neck. Hold briefly and then, inhaling, roll back again until your forehead touches the floor. Rock back and forth slowly, 20 times. Note how you stretch and release the head and neck muscles. Do this in place of the Moon.* CAUTION *Avoid if you have neck problems or neck pain.*

Epilepsy

Like a computer, your nerves and brain work through tiny electrical pulses. And, just as in a computer, a "short-circuit" occurs if the intensity of these pulses is not controlled. This happens during an epileptic seizure; here, a sudden surge of electrical discharges from the brain shocks the entire nervous system. A minor event briefly alters consciousness, and involves uncontrolled movements and speech, and visual and aural impressions. A major event entails temporary loss of consciousness, with stiffening of the whole body and rhythmic movements of the limbs and tongue. Normal consciousness soon returns, but brain damage, even death, can result if seizures are frequent or prolonged.

The treatment for epilepsy is medication that controls the seizures but, since their frequency is increased by stress and hyperventilation, yoga has a vital supporting role. It trains you not to hyperventilate, and reduces the frequency of seizures. This may enable your doctor to reduce your medication and allow you to avoid its adverse long-term effects.

FROM THE BASIC SESSION
● Emphasize: *Backward Bend; Shoulderstand; Alternate-nostril Breathing.*
○ Avoid: *Cat Stretch; Rabbit Breathing; Rapid Abdominal Breathing.*
FROM THE AILMENTS SECTION
⊕ Add: *Neck-rolling (p.83).*

Multiple Sclerosis (MS)

The cause of this disease is, as yet, unknown – other than that it attacks the nervous system. Over the years, it slowly and progressively takes away the use of the muscles, limbs, and face, and sometimes causes blindness. And since there is no medical cure, sufferers are faced with the prospect of an ever-worsening condition. Understandably, depression is often an additional problem.

If you suffer from MS, yoga can give you courage and the power to utilize whatever residual muscular capacity you have left. This is often greater than is realized, for when one group of muscles is incapacitated, another group can usually take over. Many people with MS, who thought they would be confined to wheelchairs for life, have been able to walk and resume former activities through yoga. Though retraining the body to do this is not easy, deep relaxation, *pranayama*, meditation, and movement exercises can be effective. Deeper changes in the nervous system, through regular *pranayama* and meditation, may also delay further degeneration. Even when the condition becomes very severe, yoga can help you learn to accept life as it comes through *Meditation* (p. 40), *Happiness Analysis* (p. 13), and *Emotion Culturing* (p. 41).

FROM THE BASIC SESSION
● Emphasize: *Relaxation; Pranayama; Meditation; Emotion Culturing.*
FROM THE AILMENTS SECTION
⊕ Add: *Passive Loosening (pp. 49–51).*

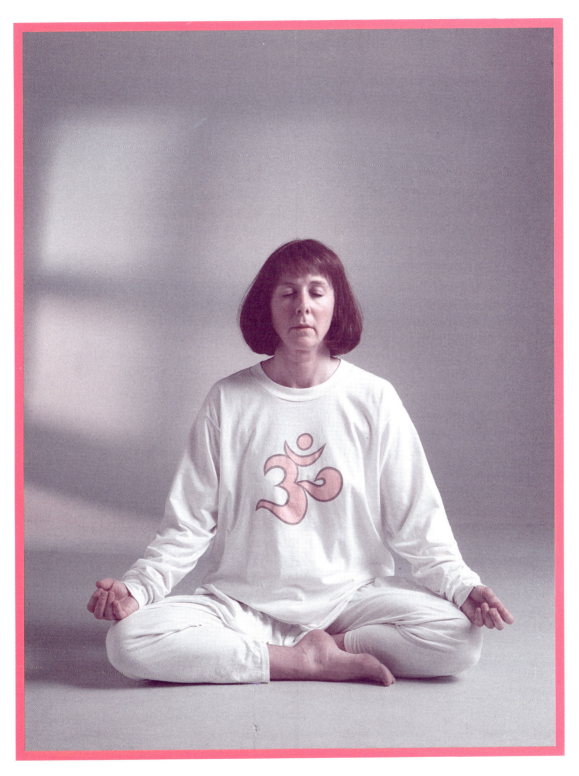

THE MEDITATION POSE

ANKIETY

Anxiety is a natural and useful response that mobilizes us to anticipate and meet danger, distress, or future problems. But too much anxiety can be a hindrance, while chronic anxiety spreads tension and apprehension to all aspects of your life. In this state, your mind becomes overactive, making you restless and unable to concentrate. It may overstimulate your autonomic nerves as well, leading to symptoms such as sweating, trembling, a dry mouth, and many others. And it can create excessive energy that makes you talk too much or cry for no reason.

A daily yoga session will help you overcome excessive anxiety, but you need to keep practising for many months to prevent a relapse. If you feel restless before your session, use up your excess energy through active exercises before you attempt *Relaxation* (p. 37), *Pranayama* (pp. 38–9), or *Meditation* (p. 40), or even the *Asanas* (pp. 26–35). Practise the exercises in *Before You Start* (pp. 20–5) for many days if necessary, until you have slowed down and can concentrate enough for the calmer practices. If you tire easily, do two or three short sessions each day, rather than one long session. Also try to cut down on cigarettes, tea, coffee, and alcohol.

FROM THE BASIC SESSION
● Emphasize: *Before You Start; Relaxation; Pranayama; Meditation; Emotion Culturing.*

DEPRESSION

We have all, at times, felt sad or miserable – and we have all had to deal with grief or disappointments. But depression is not simply a reaction to unpleasant experiences. In yogic terms it is a state in which excess energy is trapped inside us and packed down, leading to lethargy and despair. During depression, sadness is chronic and severe, sleep is disturbed, and we feel constantly tired. A general lack of enthusiasm decreases our capacity for enjoyment and our ability to work.

At first, it may be hard to counteract this feeling of hopelessness and lethargy in order to start practising yoga. But once you begin, it becomes progressively easier. The yogic therapy is to give small stimulations to bring out the suppressed energy, followed by deep relaxation to calm it down. Do a *Nasal Wash* (p. 65) every morning, and practise *Rapid Abdominal Breathing* (p. 39) before your daily session and up to four times during the day. Do at least three rounds of *Sun Salute* (pp. 24–5) before moving on to the *Asanas* (pp. 26–35). Do these much more quickly than usual, and practise *QRT* for three minutes after each group.

When you feel more collected, start cultivating yogic attitudes (p. 41) to help you improve your perspective on life.

FROM THE BASIC SESSION
● Emphasize: *Before You Start; Sun Salute; Sectional Breathing; Rapid Abdominal Breathing; Emotion Culturing.*
○ Avoid: *Meditation.*

ADDICTION

Any habit that you cannot control and have become dependent upon, could be regarded as an addiction. There are many things that can lead to compulsive dependency; these include alcohol, tobacco, and many drugs, but also many quite common substances such as tea, coffee, or chocolate. Some of these are not dangerous in small amounts but many others are much more sinister – either because they are more harmful, or else because it is harder to stop using them. As well as producing dependency by giving pleasure, many substances also produce physical dependency by changing your body chemistry and setting up self-reinforcing loops. You need more and more of them to satisfy your craving and get withdrawal symptoms when you try to stop using them.

Yoga can help you break addictive loops by slowing you down, reducing the withdrawal symptoms, and giving inner mastery, making it easier for you to resist the lure of the addictive activity. Yogic attitudes help you attain a positive sense of health, self-confidence, and the courage to face the world and overcome the guilt feelings that often follow recovery.

At first emphasize yoga practices that involve movement. Do the *Asanas* (pp. 26–35) more quickly than usual, stopping after every group of *asanas* for three or four minutes of *QRT* (p. 37). When you have learned *Rapid Abdominal Breathing* (p. 39), practise three rounds of it before you start your daily session, and also several times during the day. Also practise *Yoga Nidra* (p. 59), and make it your resolution to stop the addiction.

FROM THE BASIC SESSION
● Emphasize: *Before You Start; Sectional Breathing; Rapid Abdominal Breathing.*
FROM THE AILMENTS SECTION
⊕ Add: *Worry-beads Meditation (below).*

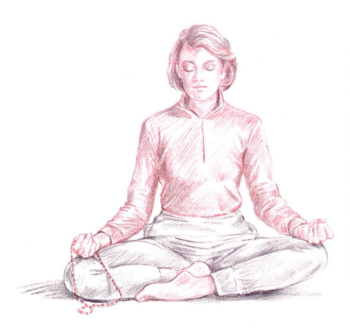

Worry-Beads Meditation *Make or buy a necklace with 108 round beads and one marker bead that you can identify by touch. Hold the marker in your dominant hand, as shown, and sit in a meditation pose (p. 40) with your eyes closed. Choose a word that has a positive meaning for you and is easy to say, such as "OM" or "GOD", and silently repeat this, moving along one bead every time you do so. Stop when you reach the marker. Ignore stray thoughts; just repeat the word without becoming anxious. Practise this exercise instead of Meditation.*

EYES

Our eyes are the most sophisticated sense organs in our bodies. They contain lenses, muscle systems, and tiny light receptors that allow us to see the world we live in; a world of colour, movement, and almost infinite distance. Yet increasingly often in these days of high stress, television, and computers we find that our vision is impaired.

The 20th century has brought us great benefits, yet the hectic pace of modern life imposes a great burden on our eyes. Visual display screens, pollution, and stress can all cause eye strain. This tends to precipitate the development of refraction errors (such as short- and long-sightedness and astigmatism), glaucoma, and allergic eye inflammations.

You are far from helpless to prevent such disorders, however. If you take conscious care of your eyes you can considerably reduce eye strain and limit the damage it causes. The yoga method of eye therapy allows you to help yourself holistically, by combining general relaxation to reduce stress with specific eye exercises. This can both arrest the rate of deterioration and bring lasting improvement to already existing eye problems.

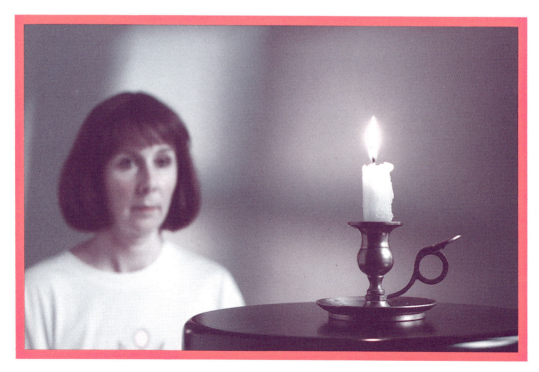

CANDLE GAZING

EYE PROBLEMS

Relaxation is the key to yogic therapy for eye problems. Your ability to see clearly in different directions, at different distances, and at different intensities of light is due to the many eye muscles. Like other muscles, these react to stress by becoming chronically overcontracted. This causes eye strain, which can contribute to many eye problems.

Refraction errors, which result from physical defects in the eyes, can be made worse by eye strain. Here, the overcontraction of the eye muscles impairs focussing and distorts the shape of the eye ball. Other eye problems (p. 88) are also made worse.

General relaxation and yogic eye exercises help to reduce strain and also build up the stamina of eye muscles. *Asanas* that act on the neck or change blood pressure to the head reduce tensions, and cleansing practices, such as the *Nasal Wash*, relieve pressure from the sinuses. *Palming* (p. 90) relaxes the eyes locally and *Candle Gazing* (p. 90) stimulates and relaxes the eyes, as well as steadying the mind. The *Focussing Exercises* (pp. 90-1) train the eyes and improve your ability to make visual adjustments. This helps you if you have to read a lot, or work at a VDU. Defocussing exercises (p. 90) help to expand your mental as well as visual awareness.

To help refractive errors you can apply the following techniques throughout the day: relax while reading under conditions that normally cause eye strain, such as at a VDU or in a noisy room; sometimes, try to decipher small print without glasses – focus on the individual letters and words and relax the eyes through *Palming* after each line; practise *Recollection* and *Dwelling In Silence* (p. 41) at intervals throughout the day.

For all eye problems, practise eye splashing (p. 91) and the *Nasal Wash* (p. 65) in the mornings and evenings. Release eye tension by blinking, looking away, *Palming*, or eye splashing. If you are aiming to treat only eye problems, you can omit the *Basic Session* and instead follow the *Special Eye Session* shown in the table below. First remove glasses or lenses. *Emphasize* eye splashing if you have a cataract and *avoid* inverted *asanas* if you have a tendency to detached retina.

SPECIAL EYE SESSION		
Exercise	Page	Time
1. Candle Gazing	90	10 minutes
2. Focussing Exercises	90-1	10 minutes
3. Forced Alternate-nostril Breathing	70	2 minutes
4. Hands-to-feet Pose	27	3 minutes
5. Backward Bend	28	2 minutes
6. Moon	33	3 minutes
7. Crocodile	30	2 minutes
8. Cobra	29	2 minutes
9. Deep Relaxation Technique	37	5 minutes
10. Alternate-nostril Breathing	39	3 minutes
11. Folded-tongue Breathing	39	2 minutes
12. Sounds Breathing	39	2 minutes

Candle-gazing *Sit comfortably, with an erect, unsupported spine. Place a candle, or an oil lamp at eye level, about 1m (3ft) away, and gaze at the gently glowing flame without blinking for 10 seconds; then, palm for 30 seconds, observing the flame's after-image. Next, gaze with one eye at a time, and finally, focus both eyes on the flame but turn your head from side to side. Repeat three times, gazing for 10, 20, then 30 seconds at first. Add 10 seconds each week, until you are gazing for one, two, and three minutes. Always palm in between gazing to avoid eyestrain. Ignore the irritation of the eyes. As your gaze becomes steady, your mind will become single-pointed.*

Palming *Sit comfortably and rub the palms of your hands together rapidly. Cup your hands over your closed eyes, sealing out all light. Tilt your head forward and rest your elbows on a table or on your knees. Relax like this for 20 seconds. Be aware of any after-images or visual sensations. If your hands are cold, warm them in hot water before starting. Palming can relieve eyestrain during the day and after the more strenuous eye exercises.*

FOCUSSING EXERCISES

The four exercises that follow act to exercise the muscles in your eyes. In the same way as a weight-lifter trains to lift ever-heavier weights, these exercises train your eye muscles, and also increase their stamina and their ability to make adjustments in focussing.

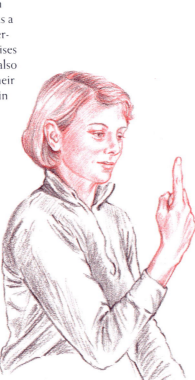

1 Centre Gazing *Touch the point between your eyebrows with your forefinger. Feel the touch. Slowly draw your finger away from you, in a straight line, until your arm is fully extended, and focus on the middle part of your forefinger as it moves. After a few seconds, slowly bring your finger back until it touches the original point. Palm, then repeat the above sequence, but this time, using the tip of your nose as a starting point. Palm again, then move on to 2.*

2 Shoulder Gazing *Extend your right arm in front of you, with your thumb pointing up. Focus on the mid point of your thumb. Slowly move your arm to the right, keeping it level, and follow the mid point of the thumb with your eyes. Go as far as you can without turning your head and then hold that position for 10 to 30 seconds. Slowly come back to the front. Palm, and repeat the sequence for the left. Palm again, and move on to 3.*

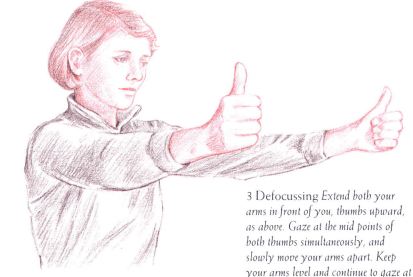

3 Defocussing *Extend both your arms in front of you, thumbs upward, as above. Gaze at the mid points of both thumbs simultaneously, and slowly move your arms apart. Keep your arms level and continue to gaze at both thumbs without turning your head. Go as far as you can without losing sight of either thumb. Hold this position for about one minute, then, slowly return to the original position. Palm and move on to 4.*

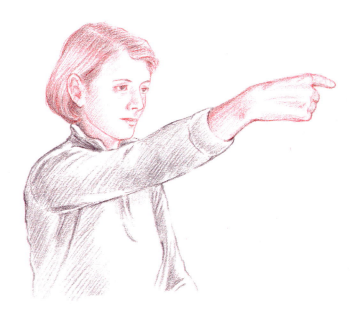

4 Up and Down Gazing *Extend your right arm and point your fore-finger to the left. Focus on the mid point of your finger as you slowly raise your arm, but don't move your head. Go as far as you can without losing sight of it. Hold for 30 seconds. Lower it to eye level and then palm. Repeat, but now focus below eye level. Do both five times alternately, then palm for one minute.*

WATER TREATMENT

This acts on the tissues and nearby sinuses. Bend over a basin of cold water and splash water into your open eyes. Then, fill an eye cup, place it over your right eye, and tilt your head back. Keep your eyelid open and roll your eye around. Repeat with your left eye. For cataracts, practise eye-cupping at least twice for each eye, three times a day (before breakfast, lunch, and supper).

91

INDEX

Bold type indicates main entry.
Italic indicates illustrations or
photographs.

AUTHORS' ACKNOWLEDGEMENTS
We thank members of the Vivekananda Kendra Yoga
Research Foundation, who helped develop the
system of yoga therapy in this book, John Blackwood
for contributing to the writing, and Jennie Elston for
discussions on yoga practices.

RESOURCES

Finding a Yoga Teacher

Try to find a yoga teacher, in addition to using this
book, who will help you learn the practices
correctly. Most teachers of *hatha yoga*, or "body"
yoga, will be able to guide you through the *asanas*,
but only some will be familiar with *pranayama* or
meditation. Standards of yoga teaching vary greatly
and it is important to choose your teacher carefully.
The organizations listed below will be able to
provide you with further information, such as lists
of yoga organizations and teachers in your area,
recent developments in research, and more
advanced yoga techniques. *Yoga Journal* and *Yoga
and Health* are also useful sources of information on
these subjects.

Organizations

Vivekananda Kendra Yoga Research Foundation,
37 IV Main Road, Malleswaram, Bangalore
560003, India.
International headquarters of the Vivekananda
Kendra Yoga Research Foundation.

Information on yoga therapy and training.
Yoga Biomedical Trust, 156 Cockerell Road,
Cambridge, CB4 3RZ, UK. Fax: 0223 313587.
Information on yoga organizations worldwide. For
USA write to: c/o 4150 Tivoli Avenue, Los
Angeles, CA 90066, USA.
Himalayan Institute of Yoga, Science, and
Philosophy, RR 1, Box 400, Honesdale, PA 18431.
For research and advanced yoga practice.
Unity in Yoga, 14426 NE 16th Place, Belleview,
Washington 98007, USA. In touch with yoga
organizations in North and South America.
International Yoga Teachers Association and Yoga
for Health Foundation, 23 Morgan Street,
Thornleigh, NSW 2120, Australia. Information on
selected yoga organizations and teaching centres.

Audio and Video Cassettes

A list of available cassettes and their sources of
supply can be obtained from most of the above
organizations, and the Yoga Biomedical Trust does
a comprehensive list for around the world. The
yoga magazines listed below are also often a useful
source of such information.

BOOKS AND PERIODICALS

Balaskas, Janet, *Natural Pregnancy*, Sidgwick & Jackson Ltd,
UK, 1990; Interlink, USA, 1990; Simon & Schuster,
Australia, 1990. Holistic methods, including yoga, to
enhance pregnancy and overcome its problems.

Chaitow, Leon, *Clear Body, Clear Mind*, Unwin Hyman,
UK, 1990; Viking O'Neil, Australia, 1990; and as *The
Body/Mind Purification Program*, Simon & Schuster, USA,
1990. How to cleanse the body of toxins.

Gharote, M L and Lockhart, Maureen (Eds.), *The Art of
Survival: a guide to yoga therapy*, Unwin Paperbacks, London
and Sydney, 1987. Reflections on the nature of yoga
therapy and its place in modern culture.

Iyengar, B K S, *Light on Yoga*, Shocken Books, New York,
1985. In depth instructions on *asanas*.

Monro, Robin, Ghosh, A K, and Kalish, Daniel, *Yoga
Research Bibliography*, Yoga Biomedical Trust, Cambridge,
1989. Key to research on yoga and health. Available from
Yoga Biomedical Trust.

Nagendra, H R and Nagarathna, R, *A New Light for
Asthmatics*, Vivekananda Kendra YOCTAS, Kanyakumari,
South India, 1986. Full account of practices given in this
book, as applied to bronchial asthma. Available from
Yoga Biomedical Trust.

Sivananda Yoga Centre, *The Book of Yoga*, Ebury Press,
London, 1983; and as *The Sivananda Companion to Yoga*,
Simon & Schuster, USA, 1983. Covers most of the
practices in this book, as well as other aspects of yoga.
Though different from the Vivekananda method, this is a
good source for further techniques.

Stanway, Penny, *Diet for Common Ailments*, Sidgwick &
Jackson Ltd, UK, 1989; Collins, Australia, 1989; and as
Foods for Common Ailments, Simon & Schuster, USA, 1989.
How to modify your diet to improve common ailments
and maintain your health.

Thomas, Sara, *Massage for Common Ailments*, Sidgwick &
Jackson Ltd, UK, 1989; Simon & Schuster, USA, 1989;
Collins, Australia, 1989. How to use touch as a healing
technique for many common disorders.

Worthington, Vivian, *A History of Yoga*, Arcana, New
York, 1982. Puts yoga into a broad, international
perspective.

Yoga Journal, 2054 University Avenue, Berkeley, CA
94704, USA. Bimonthly magazine covering a broad range
of topics.

Yoga and Health, 21 Caburn Crescent, Lewes, East Sussex,
BN7 1NR, UK. Monthly magazine covering a broad
range of topics.

Also originated by Gaia Books:

AROMATHERAPY FOR COMMON AILMENTS by Shirley Price
DIET FOR COMMON AILMENTS by Penny Stanway
MASSAGE FOR COMMON AILMENTS by Sara Thomas
CLEAR BODY CLEAR MIND by Leon Chaitow
THE BOOK OF MASSAGE by Lucy Lidell
THE BOOK OF YOGA by Lucy Lidell
THE SENSUAL BODY by Lucy Lidell
THE BOOK OF STRESS SURVIVAL by Alex Kirsta
THE MIND GYMNASIUM by Denis Postle
THE WAY OF HARMONY by Howard Reid
NATURAL MEDICINE FOR CHILDREN by Julian Scott
THE COMPLETE NEW HERBAL by Richard Mabey
GREEN INHERITANCE by Anthony Huxley
THE NATURAL HOUSE BOOK by David Pearson